Children's Costume

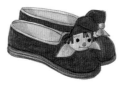

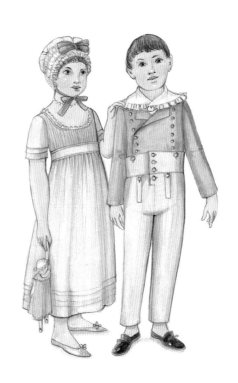

Children's Costume

The Complete Historical Sourcebook

John Peacock

with 1,045 illustrations,
730 in color

Thames & Hudson

For Madeleine and Elliot Simmonds and Jonty Peacock

p. 1 Slippers, *c.* 1951; see p. 120.
p. 2 4-year-old girl and 5-year-old boy, *c.* 1800; see p. 14.
p. 3 8-year-old girl and 12-year-old girl, 1850–74; see p. 155.
p. 6 9-year-old Egyptian princesses, *c.* 1360 BC.

First published in 2009 in hardcover in the United States of America by
Thames & Hudson Inc., 500 Fifth Avenue, New York, New York 10110

thamesandhudsonusa.com

Library of Congress Catalog Card Number 2009901945

ISBN 978-0-500-51488-7

Printed and bound in China by SNP Leefung Printers Limited

Contents

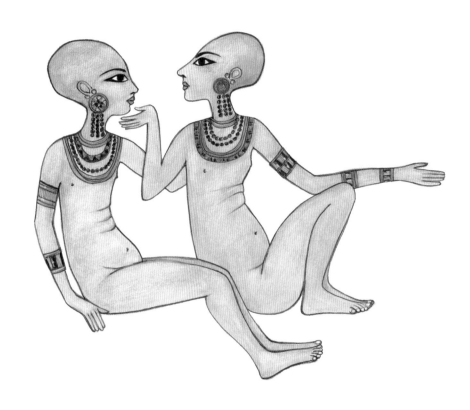

Introduction

Children's Costume follows the history of children's fashions from ancient times to the present day, covering roughly 4,000 years and several cultures. My main purpose in researching and compiling this book has been to create an accessible visible chronology of the evolution of fashionable clothes worn by girls and boys, showing as many styles as possible and concentrating on those that I consider to be the most representative of each period and of the greatest interest to the designer, student, collector and non-specialist enthusiast to whom this book is directed.

Within such a long timespan some problems of terminology and classification have obviously arisen. For those archaic, but historically accurate, expressions that may cause confusion to the non-specialist, I have substituted modern terms, particularly with regard to fabric. I am well aware of the dangers of over-simplification, but hope that the terms I have substituted will help today's reader more easily understand.

The book is divided into six parts, of sixteen pages each. The end of each section is followed by eight pages of schematic drawings, accompanied by detailed descriptions of each outfit. The examples presented are, in the main, clothes worn by middle- and upper-class children, until the second decade of the twentieth century when fashionwear became accessible and more easily affordable for most classes.

From ancient times until the beginning of the eighteenth century children had been treated as miniature adults, with little or no consideration for the form or proportions of a child's body, or for the consequences on the body of a small child of corsets and stays, which were worn from an early age. Play was something that a child from a wealthy background was neither allowed nor capable of.

The first section opens with a single page devoted to the ancient world, including examples of Egyptian, Greek, Roman and Byzantine children's wear, followed by four pages covering children's costume in the West from 1250 to 1799. The remaining pages of the section are devoted to the start of nineteenth-century Western costume through to 1833, beginning with child-friendly, loose-fitting muslin dresses for girls and all-in-one cotton playsuits for little boys but ending the period with not-so-child-friendly silk taffeta dresses with boned bodices and full skirts for girls and restricting wool suits for boys.

The second section covers 1834 to 1866. The first page shows baby dresses from 1800 to 1850, worn for christenings and on other special occasions, and made from fine cotton trimmed with silk ribbon and hand-made lace. During this period and until later in the century little boys up to the age of six were dressed the same as little girls. Older boys wore checked smocks over ankle-length trousers, while older girls wore full skirts held out with stiffened petticoats, ankle-length pantalets and heelless slippers. The section ends with a page illustrating hats, caps and bonnets from 1800 to 1866.

The third section, covering 1867 to 1899, shows a page of accessories from 1867 to 1882 and continues with drawings of girls wearing knee-length velvet-trimmed dresses with bustles, fancy bonnets trimmed with feathers and ribbons, and long side-buttoned boots, while twelve-year-old boys pose in three-piece tailored wool suits and square-toed boots. The last page illustrates accessories from 1883 to 1899.

The last three sections of the book, each commencing and ending with examples of accessories, are dedicated to the twentieth and early twenty-first centuries. At the beginning of this period most young boys from well-to-do families sported a sailor suit at some time in his life, as did many girls, trading breeches for a flared skirt. In the 1920s and '30s unfitted cotton dresses with low waist sashes and Peter Pan collars were all the rage for both young and older girls, made in a variety of fabrics, patterns and colours. The 1940s saw boys wearing hand-knitted sweaters, cardigans and even swimming costumes. Young girls of the 1950s were dressed like their mothers, often in the same fabrics and complete with watered-down versions of accessories. Brighter, stronger and more vibrant colours started to appear in children's fashions of the late 1960s, with psychedelic and fluorescent patterns following in the hippy period of the '70s. The 1980s to the present have seen grown-up styles being adapted more and more for children – mini skirts and velvet slouch hats, brightly coloured tights, feather boas and sparkly knitwear, boiler suits, patterned Wellington boots, fancy waistcoats, leather jackets and the ubiquitous unisex trainers to name but a few styles.

At the end of the book are several pages which chart the development of children's costume from antiquity to the present and outline at a glance the principal changes that have taken place. Finally, a select bibliography lists those works which have been especially useful to me in compiling this survey and will hopefully assist those who wish to take their studies further.

1500 BC—AD 400

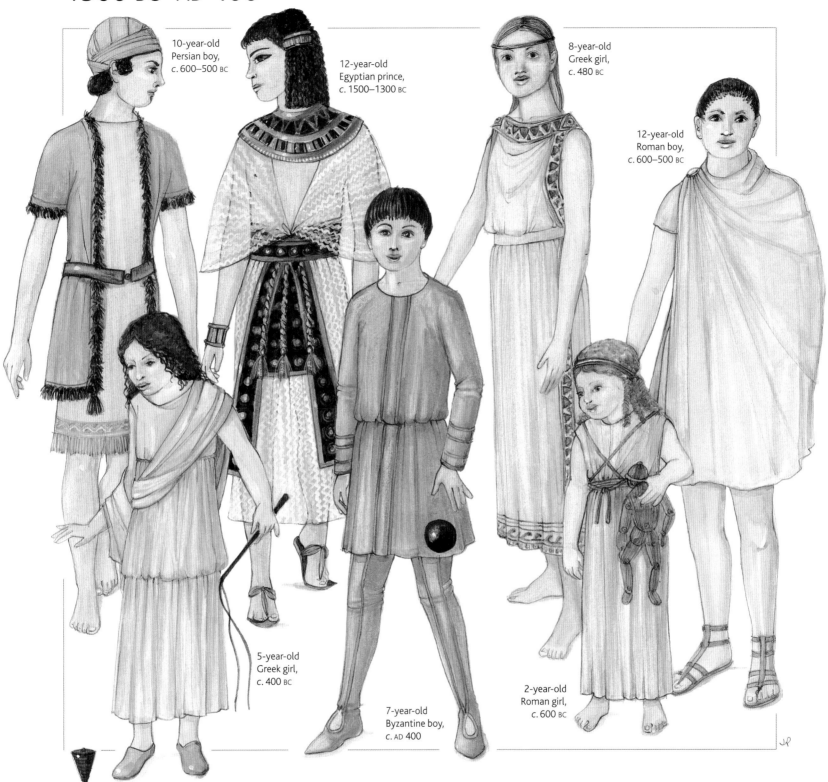

10-year-old
Persian boy,
c. 600–500 BC

12-year-old
Egyptian prince,
c. 1500–1300 BC

8-year-old
Greek girl,
c. 480 BC

12-year-old
Roman boy,
c. 600–500 BC

5-year-old
Greek girl,
c. 400 BC

7-year-old
Byzantine boy,
c. AD 400

2-year-old
Roman girl,
c. 600 BC

1250–1530

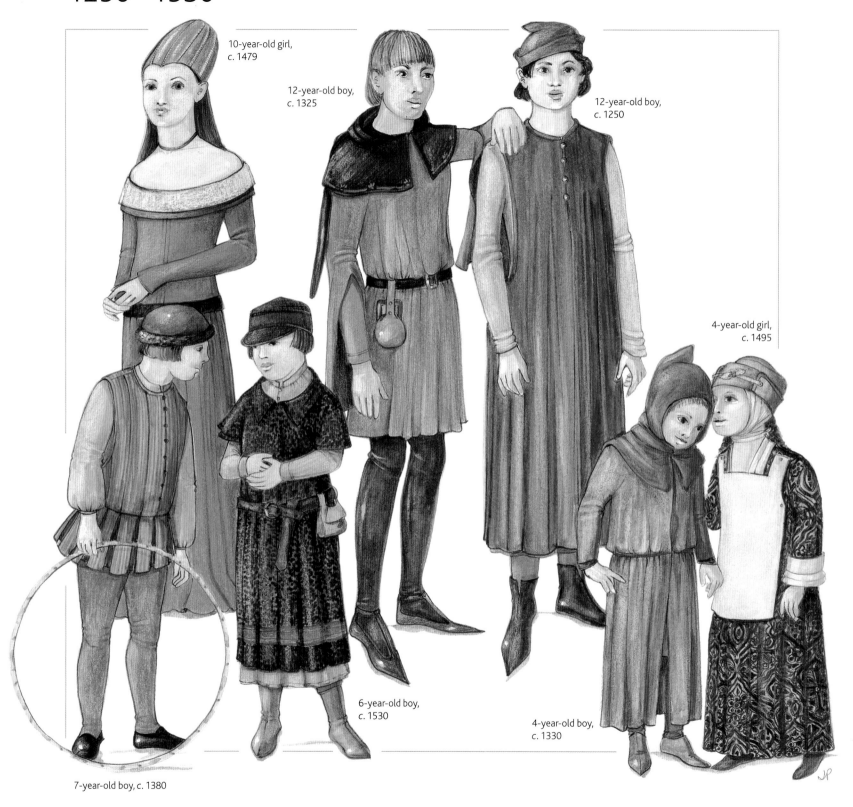

10-year-old girl, *c.* 1479

12-year-old boy, *c.* 1325

12-year-old boy, *c.* 1250

4-year-old girl, *c.* 1495

6-year-old boy, *c.* 1530

4-year-old boy, *c.* 1330

7-year-old boy, *c.* 1380

1538–1621

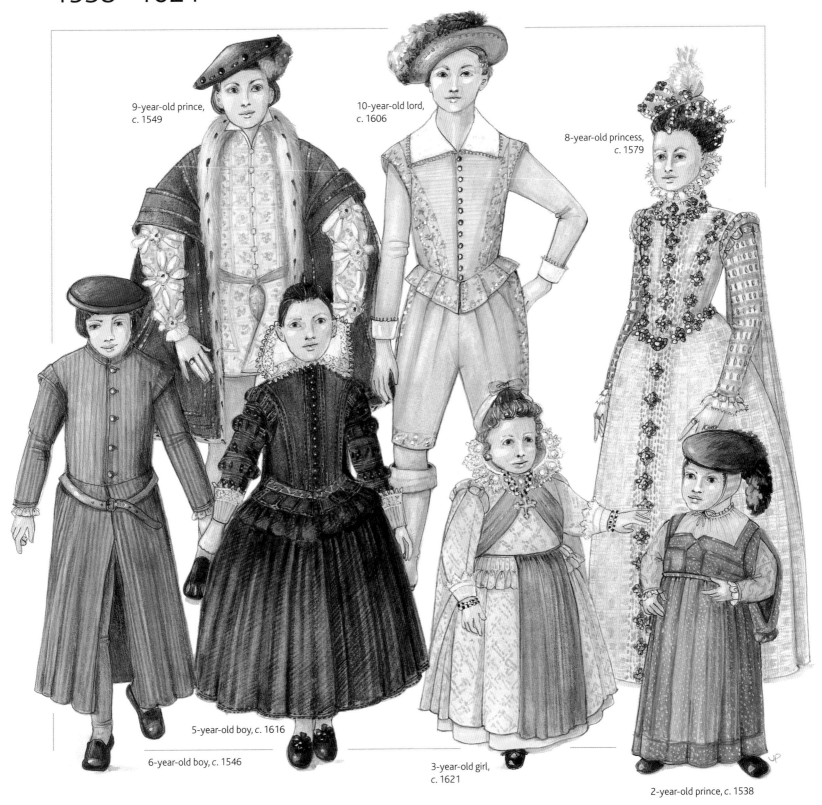

9-year-old prince, c. 1549

10-year-old lord, c. 1606

8-year-old princess, c. 1579

6-year-old boy, c. 1546

5-year-old boy, c. 1616

3-year-old girl, c. 1621

2-year-old prince, c. 1538

1635–1695

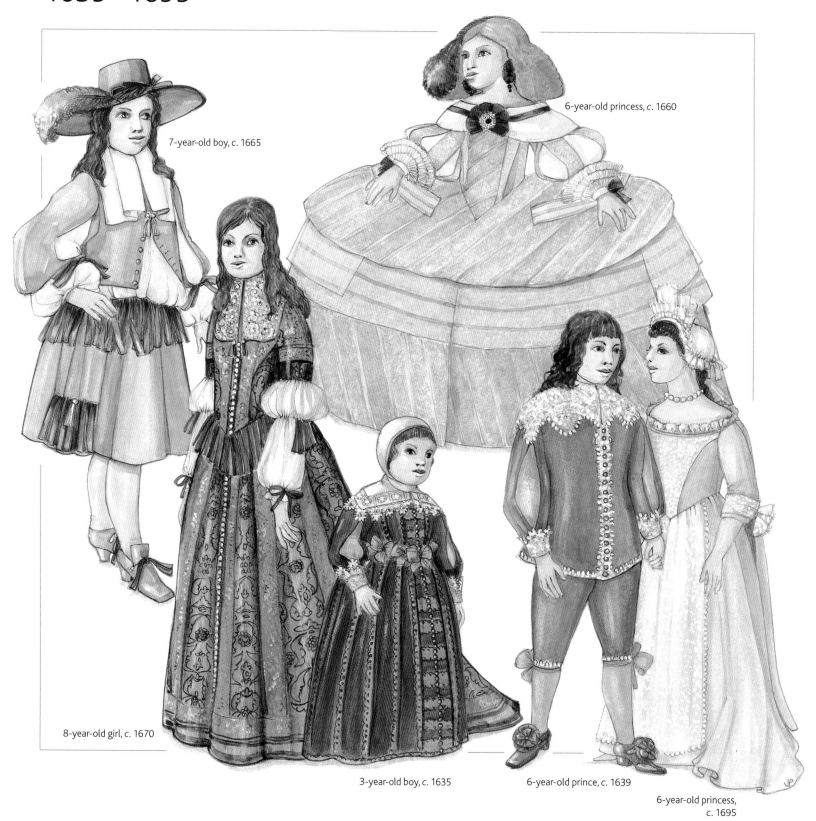

7-year-old boy, *c.* 1665

6-year-old princess, *c.* 1660

8-year-old girl, *c.* 1670

3-year-old boy, *c.* 1635

6-year-old prince, *c.* 1639

6-year-old princess, *c.* 1695

1741–1799

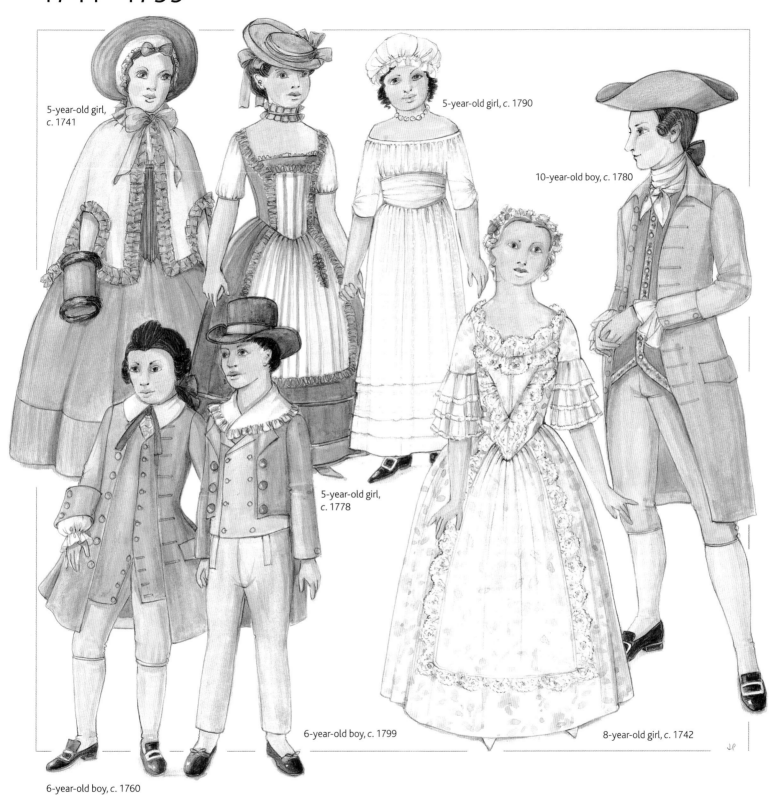

5-year-old girl, c. 1741

5-year-old girl, c. 1790

10-year-old boy, c. 1780

5-year-old girl, c. 1778

6-year-old boy, c. 1799

6-year-old boy, c. 1760

8-year-old girl, c. 1742

1800–1802

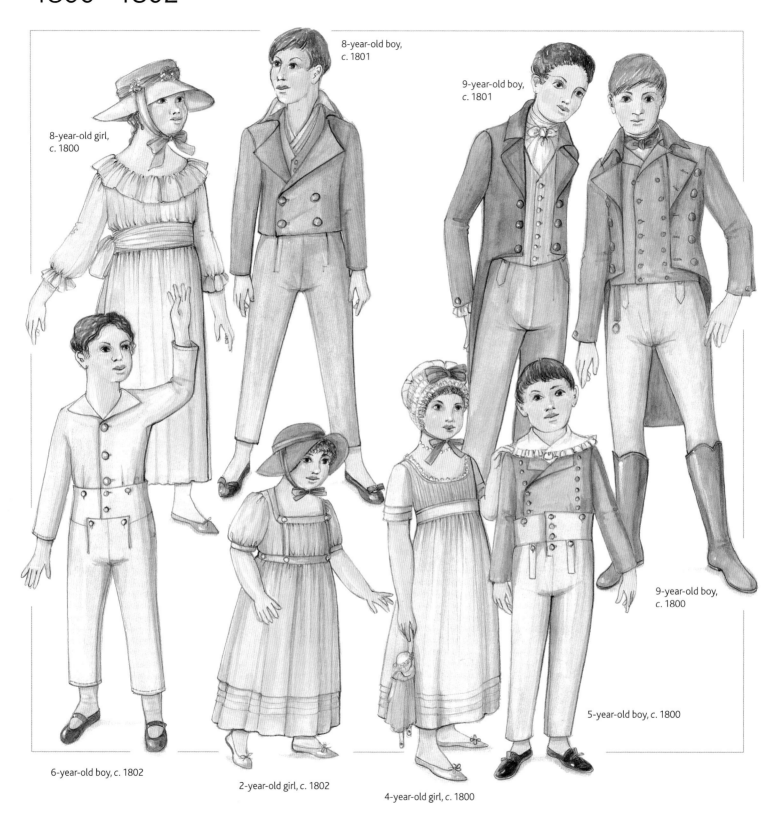

8-year-old girl, *c.* 1800

8-year-old boy, *c.* 1801

9-year-old boy, *c.* 1801

9-year-old boy, *c.* 1800

6-year-old boy, *c.* 1802

2-year-old girl, *c.* 1802

4-year-old girl, *c.* 1800

5-year-old boy, *c.* 1800

1803–1805

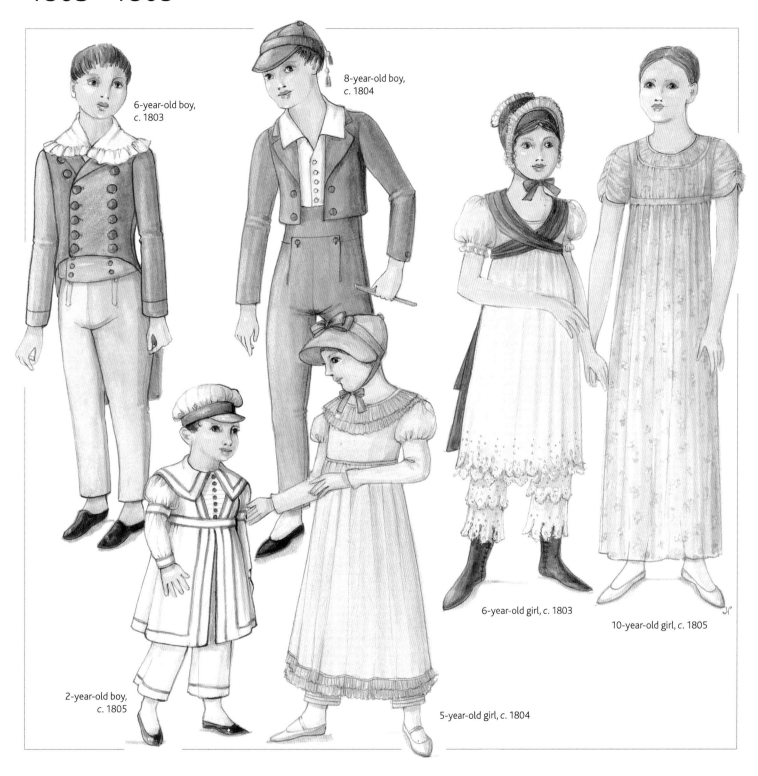

6-year-old boy, *c.* 1803

8-year-old boy, *c.* 1804

2-year-old boy, *c.* 1805

5-year-old girl, *c.* 1804

6-year-old girl, *c.* 1803

10-year-old girl, *c.* 1805

1806–1808

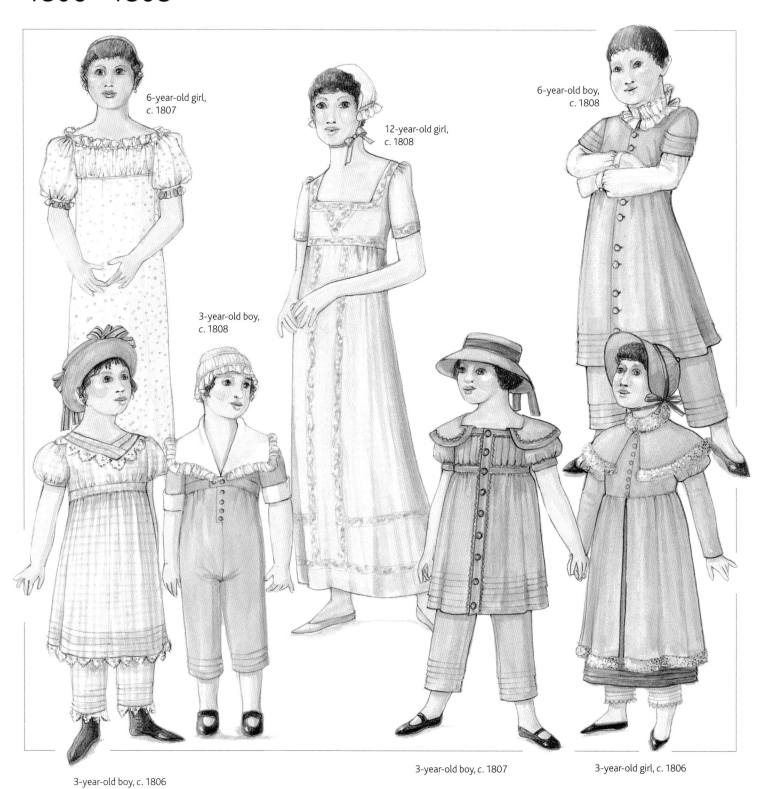

6-year-old girl,
c. 1807

12-year-old girl,
c. 1808

6-year-old boy,
c. 1808

3-year-old boy,
c. 1808

3-year-old boy, c. 1806

3-year-old boy, c. 1807

3-year-old girl, c. 1806

1809–1811

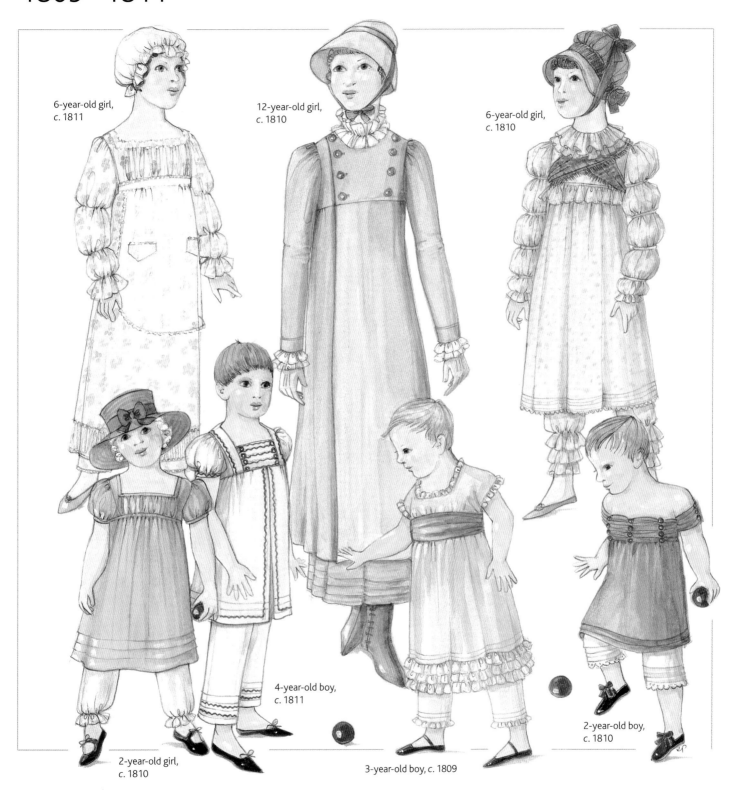

6-year-old girl,
c. 1811

12-year-old girl,
c. 1810

6-year-old girl,
c. 1810

2-year-old girl,
c. 1810

4-year-old boy,
c. 1811

3-year-old boy, c. 1809

2-year-old boy,
c. 1810

1812–1817

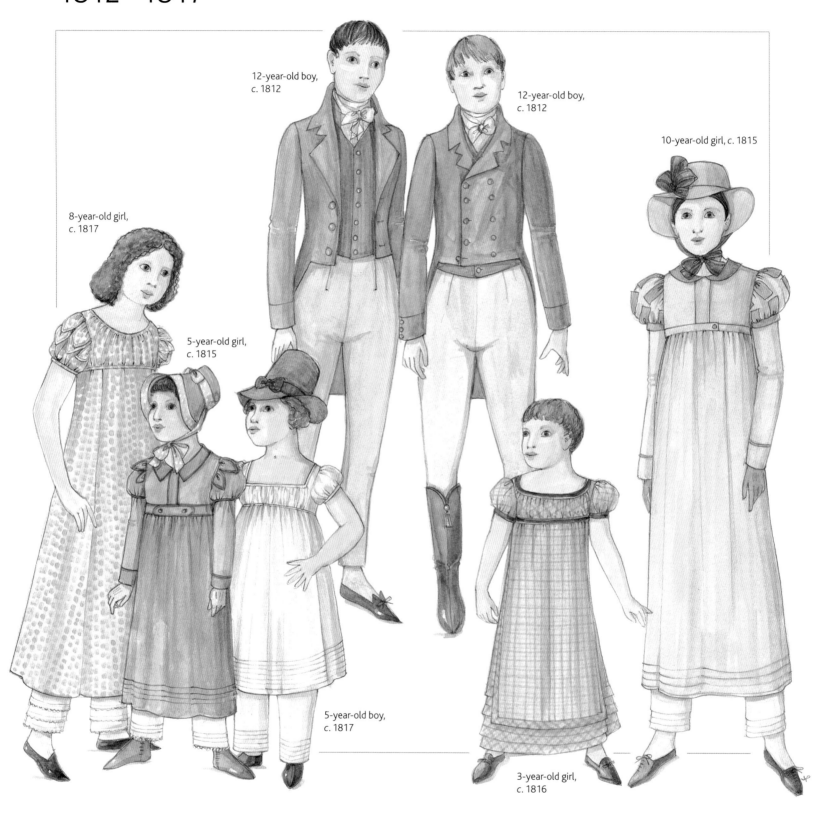

12-year-old boy, c. 1812

12-year-old boy, c. 1812

10-year-old girl, c. 1815

8-year-old girl, c. 1817

5-year-old girl, c. 1815

5-year-old boy, c. 1817

3-year-old girl, c. 1816

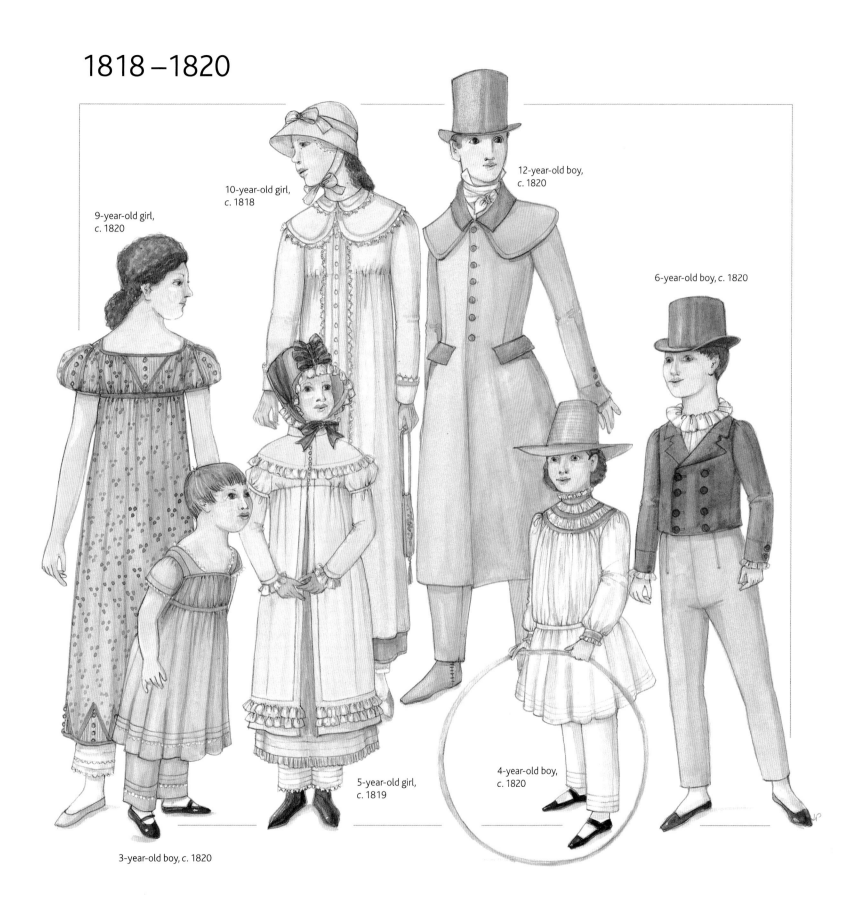

9-year-old girl, *c.* 1820

10-year-old girl, *c.* 1818

12-year-old boy, *c.* 1820

6-year-old boy, *c.* 1820

3-year-old boy, *c.* 1820

5-year-old girl, *c.* 1819

4-year-old boy, *c.* 1820

1821–1822

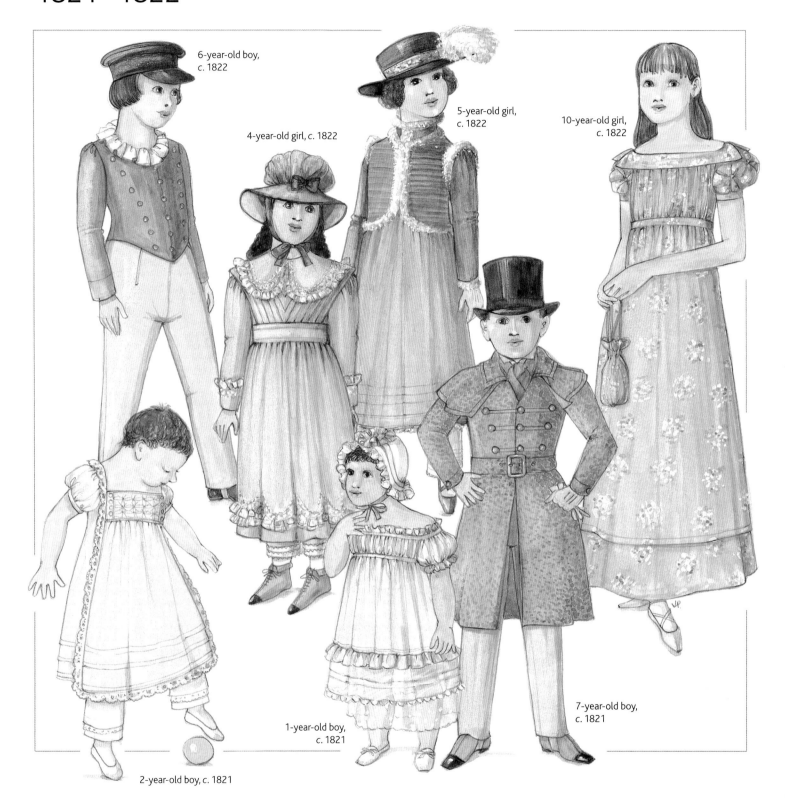

6-year-old boy,
c. 1822

4-year-old girl, c. 1822

5-year-old girl,
c. 1822

10-year-old girl,
c. 1822

2-year-old boy, c. 1821

1-year-old boy,
c. 1821

7-year-old boy,
c. 1821

1823–1825

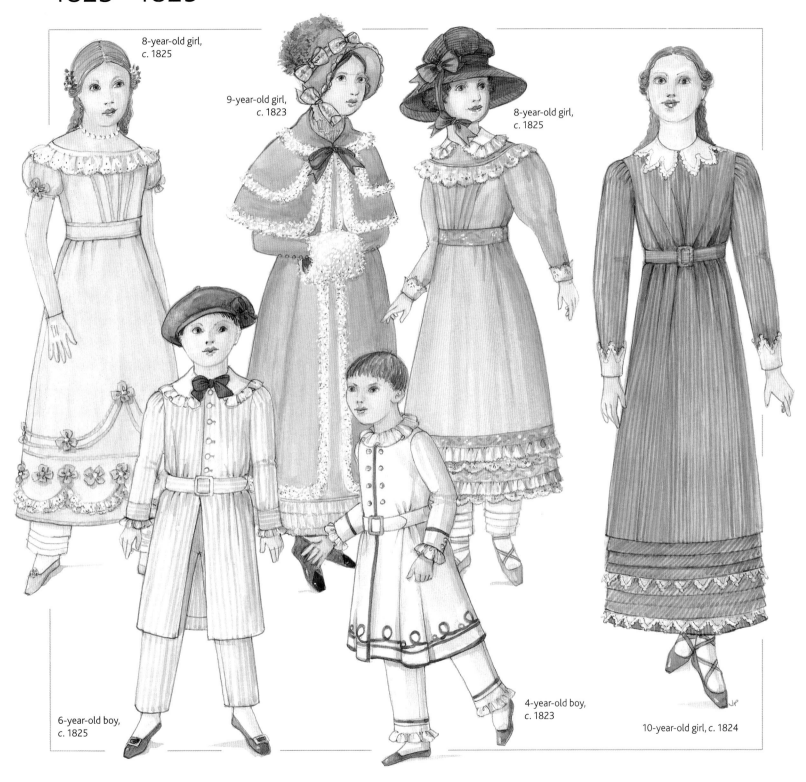

8-year-old girl, c. 1825

9-year-old girl, c. 1823

8-year-old girl, c. 1825

6-year-old boy, c. 1825

4-year-old boy, c. 1823

10-year-old girl, c. 1824

1826 –1827

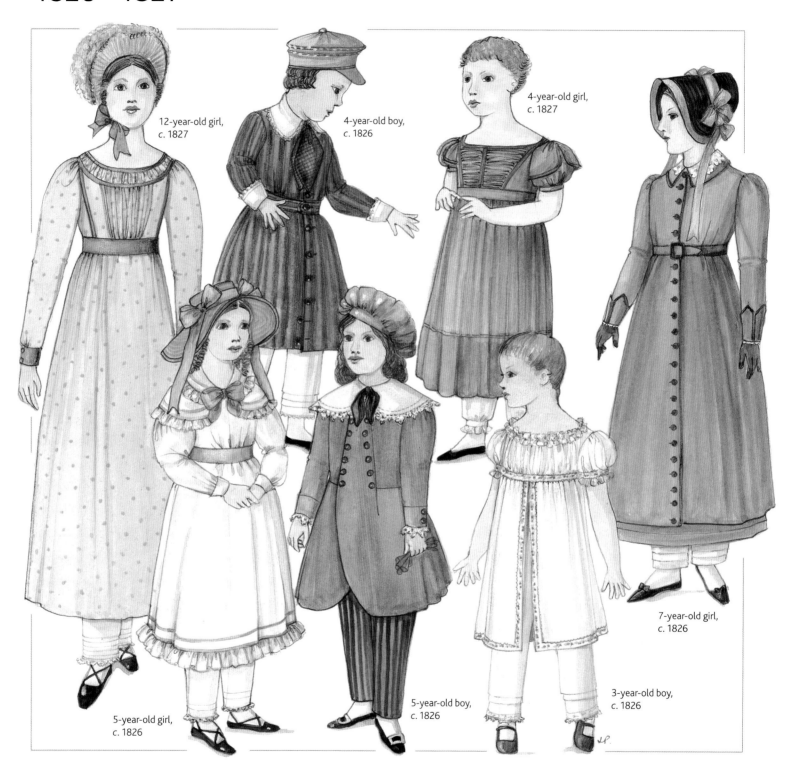

12-year-old girl,
c. 1827

4-year-old boy,
c. 1826

4-year-old girl,
c. 1827

5-year-old girl,
c. 1826

5-year-old boy,
c. 1826

3-year-old boy,
c. 1826

7-year-old girl,
c. 1826

1828 –1830

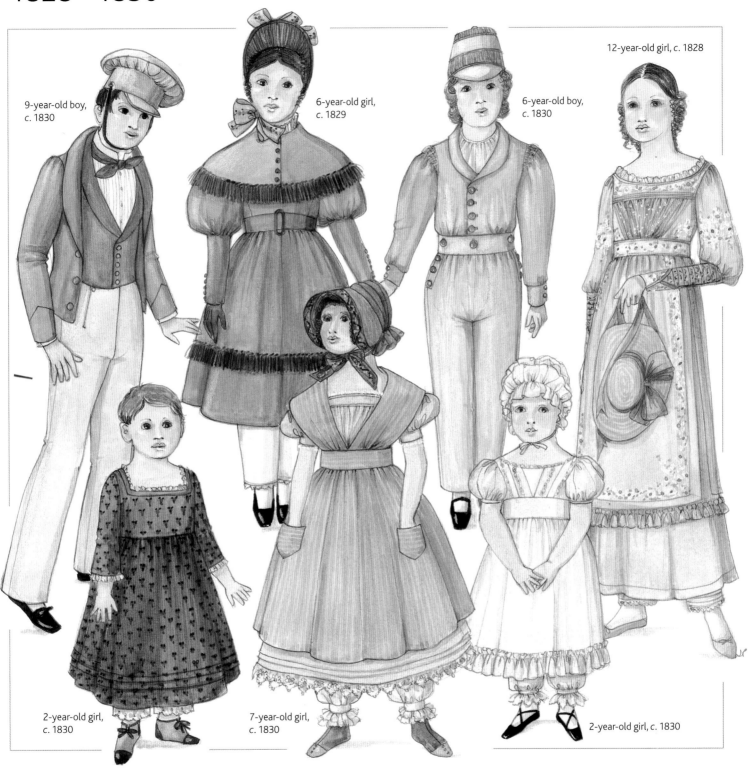

9-year-old boy, c. 1830

6-year-old girl, c. 1829

6-year-old boy, c. 1830

12-year-old girl, c. 1828

2-year-old girl, c. 1830

7-year-old girl, c. 1830

2-year-old girl, c. 1830

1831–1833

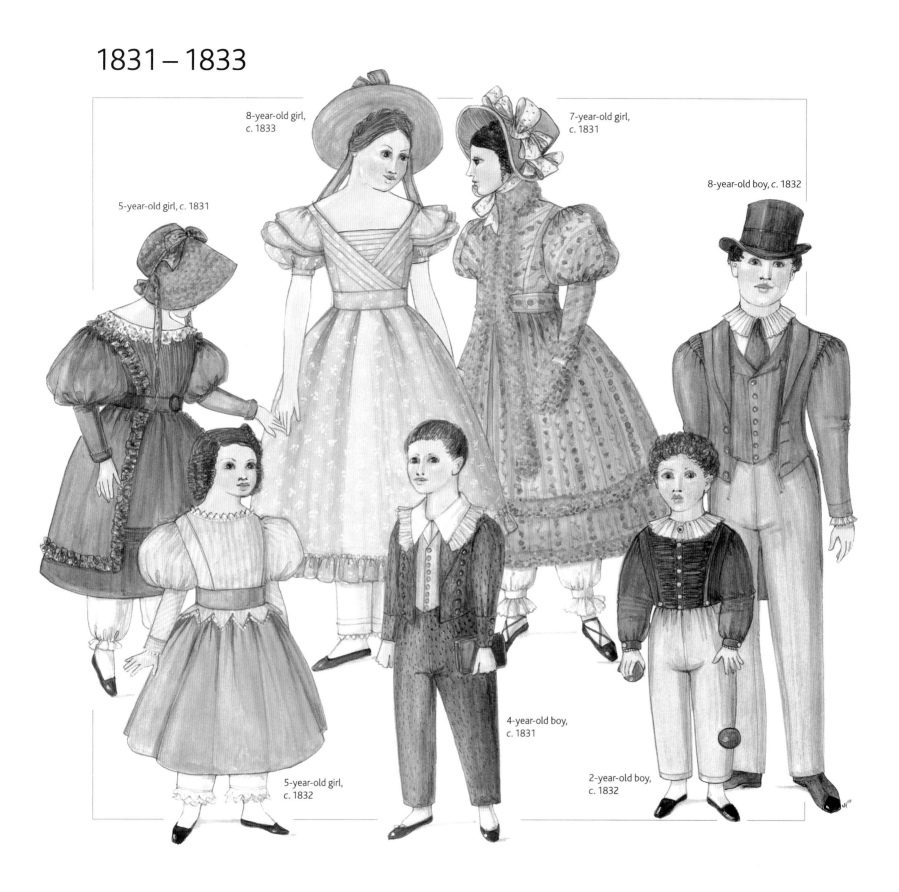

5-year-old girl, *c.* 1831

8-year-old girl, *c.* 1833

7-year-old girl, *c.* 1831

8-year-old boy, *c.* 1832

5-year-old girl, *c.* 1832

4-year-old boy, *c.* 1831

2-year-old boy, *c.* 1832

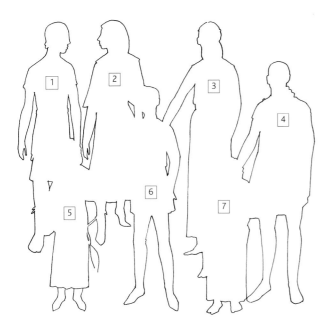

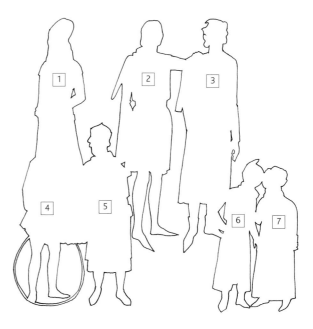

1500 BC–AD 400

1 10-year-old Persian boy, *c.* 600–500 BC. Hip-length short-sleeved wool coat with fringed edges. Knee-length undertunic with fringed and braid-trimmed hemline. Hip-level leather belt. Head bound with long continuous strip of narrow fabric. Short curly hair. 2 12-year-old Egyptian prince, *c.* 1500–1300 BC. Mid-calf-length semi-transparent pleated linen robe with no sewn seams. Large sleeve-like cape. Wide painted and jewelled waist-sash with flared trailing ends and matching loin cloth. Shoulder-wide beaded and embroidered collar, gold bracelet and matching clasp worn on one side of large elaborately curled wig. Backless sandals with coloured linings and upturned pointed toes. 3 8-year-old Greek girl, *c.* 480 BC. Simple mid-calf-length seamless tunic secured on each shoulder with a brooch pin, bloused bodice formed above wide waist-sash, open sides, wide decorative painted borders. Narrow leather head band worn above the eyebrows. Long hair with centre parting. 4 12-year-old Roman boy, *c.* 600–500 BC. Short semi-circular wool cape secured on one shoulder by large brooch pin, worn over short-sleeved tunic. Ankle-length leather strap sandals with open toes. Short cropped hair worn combed forward. 5 5-year-old Greek girl, *c.* 400 BC. Sleeveless ankle-length fine wool tunic with no sewn seams and cord belts at high waist and hip level forming bloused effect. Long fine wool shawl worn draped over one shoulder. Soft leather shoes. Long curly hair. 6 7-year-old Byzantine boy, *c.* AD 400. Collarless tunic bloused on waist above short skirt, with centre-front inset band of contrasting colour from neck to hem and two matching bands at wrist level and above on full-length sleeves. Repeated decoration on fronts of leather-soled leggings with pointed toes. Short cropped hair. 7 2-year-old Roman girl, *c.* 600 BC. Ankle-length fine wool sleeveless tunic bound on high waist and across chest with fine cord. Silver head band worn over long curly hair.

1250–1530

1 10-year-old girl, *c.* 1479. Low-necked gown with wide collar and short transparent over-collar, fitted bodice, hip-level belt and full-length circular-cut skirt. Narrow ribbon worn around throat. Tall headdress, with long hair falling loose at the back. 2 12-year-old boy, *c.* 1325. Short cape and hood with waist-length point and embroidered hem. Loose-fitting knee-length tunic with long sleeves slashed at the front from wrist to elbow level revealing long tight sleeves of contrast-coloured undertunic. Low-slung leather belt with attached leather purse. Knitted stockings. Heelless leather shoes with long pointed toes. Jaw-length hair with straight fringe. 3 12-year-old boy, *c.* 1250. Collarless mid-calf-length tunic with armholes cut away to hip level, front button fastening to chest level. Collarless undertunic with long tight sleeves. Small knitted hat with pointed crown. Knitted stockings. Heelless ankle-length leather boots with long pointed toes. 4 7-year-old boy, *c.* 1380. Short collarless and sleeveless tunic with padded bodice, front button fastening and short box-pleated skirt. Undertunic with full-length sleeves gathered into narrow cuffs. Knitted stockings. Heelless leather shoes. Small hat with fur trim. Short hair. 5 6-year-old boy, *c.* 1530. Mid-calf-length tunic with large collar, short sleeves and pleated skirt, braid trim above hem. Long undertunic with full-length tight sleeves, high round neckline and small stand-up collar. Hip-level leather belt with attached purse. Long heelless leather boots with pointed toes. Stiffened fabric hat with front peak and wide band. Short hair. 6 4-year-old boy, *c.* 1330. Short shoulder cape with pointed hood. Ankle-length tunic, open down front to hem, with narrow waist-level belt forming bloused bodice, long tight sleeves. Knee-length undertunic with long sleeves. Knitted stockings. Heelless leather shoes. 7 4-year-old girl, *c.* 1495. Ankle-length patterned gown with low square neckline, long sleeves with deep stiffened cuffs, matching apron pinned to tight bodice, pleated skirt worn over petticoats. Heelless leather shoes. Close-fitting hat with turned-up brim at back, worn with neck and chin cloths, long hair falling loose at the back.

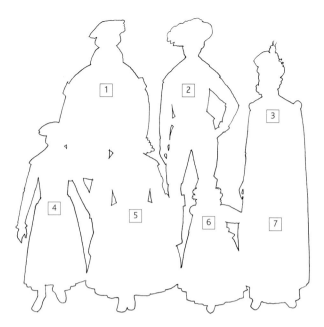

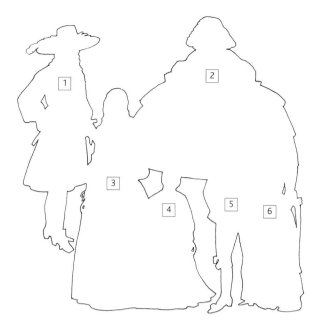

1538 – 1621

[1] 9-year-old prince, *c.* 1549. Knee-length velvet coat with deep-cuffed short sleeves, wide shoulders, ermine collar and trim. Silk undertunic with button fastening, jewelled and slashed sleeves, hip-length skirts and ribbon belt. Flat hat trimmed with large feather and decorated with jewelled brooches, matching large finger ring. Silk hose. Leather shoes with slashed blunt toes. [2] 10-year-old lord, *c.* 1606. Single-breasted silk tunic with large lace-edged collar and matching cuffs on full-length sleeves, gold embroidered lace trim on epaulettes, side fronts of fitted bodice, peplum and side seams and hems of knee-length breeches. Hat with turned-back brim, embroidered edge and large feather trim. Silk hose. Long suede boots with small heels and turned-down cuffs. [3] 8-year-old princess, *c.* 1579. Floor-length silk gown with fitted bodice, padded epaulettes, hanging sleeves and full skirt decorated with pins and brooches. Matching trim on small brimless hat and hair ornaments, high lace-edged neck ruff and cuffs on braid-trimmed full-length sleeves. Finger rings set with large jewels. [4] 6-year-old boy, *c.* 1546. Single-breasted wool coat with fitted bodice buttoned to waist, narrow stand collar, long sleeves with epaulettes and ankle-length skirts. Narrow leather belt. Flat hat with narrow brim. Knitted silk hose. Leather shoes with blunt toes. [5] 5-year-old boy, *c.* 1616. Silk gown with button-through fitted bodice, padded epaulettes, puffed and slashed sleeves, peplum above hip-level puffed section of full skirt, braided edges and trim. Lace-trimmed semi-circular collar and matching cuffs. Knitted silk hose. Leather shoes with rosettes above blunt toes. [6] 3-year-old girl, *c.* 1621. Silk gown with full-length sleeves, hanging sleeves, epaulettes and fitted bodice with contrast-colour cross-over sashes, matching apron worn above ankle-length full skirt with gathered hip detail, longer underskirt. Semi-circular lace-edged collar, matching cuffs. Gold crucifix on bead chain, matching bracelets. Small cap with bow. Leather shoes with blunt toes and ribbon ties. [7] 2-year-old prince, *c.* 1538. Full-length velvet gown with low square neckline, fur-trimmed hanging sleeves and gathered panelled skirt, gold braid edging and trim, patterned silk sleeves, collarless lace-trimmed undershirt. Brimless hat with large feather trim, worn over close-fitting bonnet. Leather shoes with blunt toes.

1635 – 1695

[1] 7-year-old boy, *c.* 1665. Short single-breasted wool jacket with large open sleeves, matching gathered knee-length breeches with looped ribbon trim at waist, outside leg and hem of shirt sleeves. Shirt with folded collar, large sleeves and full gathered bodice. Hat with high crown and wide brim with feather and looped ribbon trim. Knitted silk stockings. Leather shoes with small heels, high tongues and ribbon ties above square toes. [2] 6-year-old princess, *c.* 1660. Striped silk gown with fitted bodice, off-the-shoulder neckline with brooch and looped ribbon on centre front, matching bows on tiered pleated cuffs under large strap sleeves, exaggerated skirt worn over frame. Large earrings. Curled hair with feather decoration. [3] 8-year-old girl, *c.* 1670. Patterned silk gown with fitted bodice, cuffed elbow-length sleeves and panels of trailing skirt edged and trimmed with braids and gold lace, buttons run from under large lace collar to hem, loops of ribbon trim at waist, matching detail on long undersleeves. [4] 3-year-old boy, *c.* 1635. Full-length button-through silk gown with fronts of fitted bodice and panelled skirt edged and trimmed with gold lace and braid, matching loops and bows on waist, large lace-edged collar and cuffs on long open sleeves. Close-fitting bonnet. [5] 6-year-old prince, *c.* 1639. Single-breasted silk satin jacket with button fastening from under shoulder-wide lace collar to lace-trimmed hemline, full-length open sleeves with matching lace cuffs. Fitted knee-length breeches matching jacket fabric. Silk stockings held up by wide silk ribbon garters tied in bows on side, leather shoes with small heels and rosettes above square toes. [6] 6-year-old princess, *c.* 1695. Silk gown with low lace-edged neckline, matching front panel of fitted bodice, cuffs on three-quarter-length sleeves and decorative apron over front of long trailing skirt. Gathered cap with rows of high stiffened lace frills at the front. Short pearl necklace.

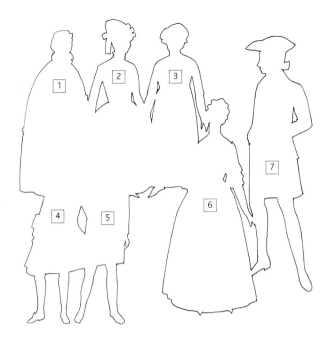

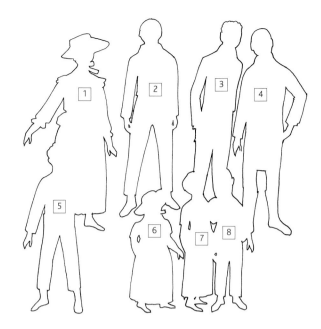

1741 – 1799

1 5-year-old girl, *c.* 1741. Silk dress with low neckline, boned bodice and ankle-length full skirt. Hip-length silk cape with frill collar, self-fabric bow-tie fastening and pleated decoration on all edges. Large straw hat worn over indoor frilled cap decorated with small bow on front. Small fur-trimmed hand muff. 2 5-year-old girl, *c.* 1778. Sleeveless silk dress with low square neckline, fitted bodice and full-length skirt, hem trimmed with ribbon, worn over chemise with short sleeves and frilled neckline. Striped silk apron with self-fabric ruched edges. Straw hat with wide brim and shallow crown, silk ribbon bow and streamer trim. Silk shoes with pointed toes. 3 5-year-old girl, *c.* 1790. Spotted fine cotton voile dress with off-the-shoulder neckline, elbow-length sleeves and ankle-length skirt gathered from under wide silk waist-sash, tucked detail above hemline. Large indoor cap with frilled edge. Short pearl necklace. Leather shoes with large buckles under high tongues, pointed toes and low heels. 4 6-year-old boy, *c.* 1760. Collarless single-breasted silk coat, cut to be worn open, buttons from neckline to hip level, tight sleeves with turned-back buttoned cuffs, full skirts, hip-level flap pockets. Single-breasted silk waistcoat. Ribbon tie under large shirt collar, ruffled front and cuffs. Knee-length breeches, buttons on side knee. Wig with side curls, back hair tied in large bow. Knitted stockings. Leather shoes with buckles under high tongues, round toes and low heels. 5 6-year-old boy, *c.* 1799. Short fine wool tail coat, cut to be worn open, narrow revers, tight sleeves. Double-breasted silk waistcoat with narrow collar. Shirt with large frill-edged collar. Felt hat with wide brim and tall crown with ribbon band. Narrow ankle-length pantaloons. Knitted stockings. Heelless leather shoes with bow trim above round toes. 6 8-year-old girl, *c.* 1742. Floor-length patterned silk dress with low lace-trimmed neckline, matching trim on fitted bodice, tiered frills on short sleeves and transparent apron over gathered skirt. Indoor cap decorated with flowers and lace frills. Silk shoes with pointed toes. 7 10-year-old boy, *c.* 1780. Single-breasted knee-length coat, cut to be worn open, tight sleeves with cuffs, hip-level flap pockets. Collarless single-breasted waistcoat with embroidered edges, matching buttons. Shirt with ruffled cuffs, worn with neck stock. Knee-length breeches, buttons on side knee. Tricorn hat. Knitted stockings. Leather shoes with buckles under high tongues, round toes and low heels.

1800 – 1802

1 8-year-old girl, *c.* 1800. Ankle-length cotton dress with low neckline edged with wide self-fabric frill, matching hems of full-length sleeves, gathered skirt from high waistline, wide contrast-colour sash tied in bow at back. Straw hat with wide brim and shallow crown decorated with ribbon and flowers, tied under chin with ribbon bow. Knitted silk stockings. Heelless slippers with pointed toes. 2 8-year-old boy, *c.* 1801. Short double-breasted fine wool jacket with wide revers, high collar and tight sleeves. Collarless single-breasted silk waistcoat, worn over cotton shirt with draped front and large collar. Ankle-length wool pantaloons with fall fronts. Knitted silk stockings. Heelless leather shoes with pointed toes. 3 9-year-old boy, *c.* 1801. Fine wool tailcoat, cut to be worn open, with wide revers, high collar and tight sleeves. Collarless single-breasted silk waistcoat, worn over shirt with frills at wrist level, matching stock. Wool pantaloons with fall fronts. 4 9-year-old boy, *c.* 1800. Double-breasted wool tailcoat with wide revers, high collar and tight sleeves open at wrist with button trim. Double-breasted silk waistcoat with small collar and revers, worn over shirt and coloured stock tied in bow. Wool pantaloons tucked into high leather boots with blunt toes and small heels. 5 6-year-old boy, *c.* 1802. Skeleton suit: single-breasted collarless cotton shirt with turned-back revers and long sleeves, buttoned at waist to ankle-length pantaloons in matching fabric. Knitted stockings. Heelless leather shoes with bar straps and blunt toes. 6 2-year-old girl, *c.* 1802. Cotton dress with low square neckline, short puff sleeves, bodice buttoned to ankle-length gathered skirt at high waist level, tucked detail above hem. Straw hat with wide brim and shallow crown, tied under chin with ribbon bow. Heelless silk shoes with pointed toes. 7 4-year-old girl, *c.* 1800. Cotton dress with low neckline, high waistline, short sleeves with tucks above hem, matching detail on gathered ankle-length skirt. Frilled and ruched bonnet trimmed with ribbon, matching bow tie under chin. Heelless silk shoes with pointed toes. 8 5-year-old boy, *c.* 1800. Double-breasted wool jacket with brass buttons, narrow revers and tight sleeves, buttoned to ankle-length wool pantaloons with fall fronts. Cotton shirt with large collar and frilled edge. Knitted silk stockings. Heelless leather shoes with blunt toes.

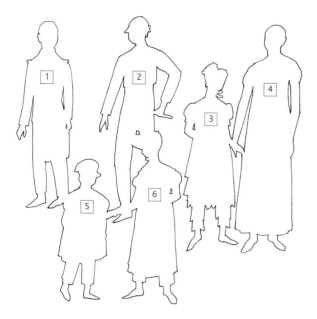

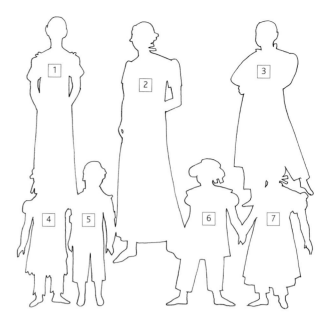

1803–1805

1 6-year-old boy, *c.* 1803. Double-breasted wool tailcoat with large buttons, tight sleeves and stitched cuffs, worn over double-breasted wool waistcoat and shirt with large frill-edged collar. Ankle-length wool pantaloons with fall fronts. Knitted stockings. Heelless leather slippers with pointed toes. 2 8-year-old boy, *c.* 1804. Short double-breasted jacket cut to be worn open, with large decorative buttons and long tight sleeves. Shirt with button fastening and open collar worn over wide revers. High-waisted ankle-length wool pantaloons with fall fronts. Knitted stockings. Heelless leather slippers with pointed toes. 3 6-year-old girl, *c.* 1803. Cotton dress with low neckline, puff sleeves and short bodice with front cross-over silk sash tied at back, eyelet embroidery around hem of short skirt, matching two-tier drawers. Taffeta bonnet with contrast-colour pleated taffeta trim on edges of tall crown and turned-up brim, ribbon trim and bow tie under chin. Heelless cloth boots with side-laced fastenings and pointed toes. 4 10-year-old girl, *c.* 1805. Fine sprigged cotton voile dress with round neckline edged with ruched detail, matching short sleeves and short bodice, ankle-length skirt gathered from under high waist-belt. Knitted silk stockings. Heelless silk slippers with pointed toes. 5 2-year-old boy, *c.* 1805. Cotton dress with short pin-tucked bodice and short puff sleeves above long cuffed sleeves, shoulder-wide collar and knee-length split skirt, with ankle-length drawers in matching fabric, braid-trimmed edges and detail. Cotton peaked cap with gathered crown and contrast-colour band. Knitted stockings. Heelless cloth slippers with pointed toes. 6 5-year-old girl, *c.* 1804. Cotton dress with short bodice, puff sleeves above long tight sleeves, wide neckline with self-fabric pleated edge, matching hem of ankle-length skirt; drawers in matching fabric. Straw bonnet with front brim and shallow crown, ribbon trim and bow tie under chin. Knitted silk stockings. Heelless silk slippers with bar straps and pointed toes.

1806–1808

1 6-year-old girl, *c.* 1807. Spotted cotton voile dress with low frill-edged neckline, matching hems of short puff sleeves, ankle-length skirt from under ruched bodice with high waist. Ribbon band worn in hair. 2 12-year-old girl, *c.* 1808. Fine cotton dress with low square neckline edged with embroidery, matching sleeves, high waist and panels of ankle-length skirt. Small frill-edged indoor bonnet with ties under chin. Knitted silk stockings. Heelless cloth shoes with pointed toes. 3 6-year-old boy, *c.* 1808. Knee-length cotton dress with front button fastening from under round neckline and short sleeves with tucks above hem, matching detail on skirt and drawers. Cotton shirt with double frill collar and long sleeves. Knitted cotton stockings. Heelless cloth shoes with pointed toes. 4 3-year-old boy, *c.* 1806. Checked cotton dress with V-shaped neckline, tucked and lace detail, matching hems of knee-length skirt and ankle-length drawers, high waist-belt, short puff sleeves. Straw hat with turned-back brim and shallow crown, looped ribbon trim. Heelless cloth ankle boots with side lacing and pointed toes. 5 3-year-old boy, *c.* 1808. Cotton combination suit: bodice with high waist joined to short pantaloons, front button fastening under large contrast-colour frill-edged collar, cuffs of short sleeves in matching colour. Ruched and frilled cotton indoor bonnet. Knitted cotton stockings. Heelless cloth shoes with buttoned bar straps and blunt toes. 6 3-year-old boy, *c.* 1807. Knee-length cotton dress with low neckline bound in contrast colour, matching wide collar, short puff sleeves, pleated bodice and button-through fastening from neck to tucked hem; drawers with matching tucked detail. Straw hat with turned-down brim, shallow crown and ribbon trim. Knitted cotton stockings. Heelless cloth shoes with buttoned bar straps and blunt toes. 7 3-year-old girl, *c.* 1806. Knee-length wool coat, front fastening under fur collar to high waist, cape and hemline trimmed with matching fur, long sleeves with puff oversleeves. Dress with tucked hemline. Drawers with tucks and lace trim. Straw bonnet with ribbon trim, bow tie under chin. Knitted silk stockings. Heelless cloth shoes with pointed toes.

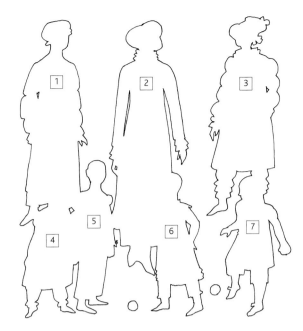

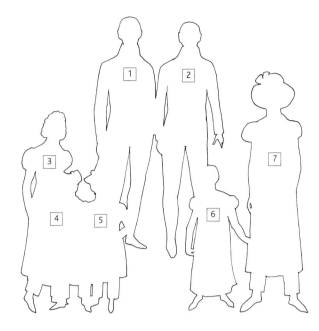

1809 – 1811

[1] 6-year-old girl, *c.* 1811. Patterned cotton dress with low neckline, short ruched bodice, three-tier puff sleeves ending in wrist frills and ankle-length skirt with ruched detail on hem; drawers in matching fabric. Dress worn with decorative transparent cotton apron with small pockets. Indoor frilled cotton cap. Knitted cotton stockings. Heelless cloth shoes with rosettes above pointed toes. [2] 12-year-old girl, *c.* 1810. Collarless mid-calf-length wool coat with high waist, double-breasted fastening, long sleeves with gathered heads and sewn cuffs, cotton ruffles at neck and wrist. Straw hat with ribbon trim and bow tie under chin. Cloth gloves. Heelless cloth ankle boots with side laces and pointed toes. [3] 6-year-old girl, *c.* 1810. Spotted cotton voile dress with five-tiered puff sleeves ending in wrist frills, matching frill at high waist and double frill at neck, knee-length skirt above drawers in matching fabric, dress worn with cashmere scarf crossed over short bodice and tied at back. Bonnet with straw brim and gathered cloth crown, looped ribbon and bow trim. Knitted cotton stockings. Heelless cloth shoes with rosette above pointed toes. [4] 2-year-old girl, *c.* 1810. Cotton dress with low square neckline, puff sleeves, ruched bodice and knee-length skirt, tucked detail around hem. Ankle-length drawers with frilled hem. Straw hat with wide brim and high crown, ribbon and bow trim. Knitted cotton stockings. Heelless leather shoes with tied bar straps and blunt toes. [5] 4-year-old boy, *c.* 1811. Cotton dress with low neckline, short bodice and puff sleeves trimmed with coloured braid, matching open skirt with tucked detail around hem and ankle-length drawers. Heelless cloth shoes with tied bar straps and blunt toes. [6] 3-year-old boy, *c.* 1809. Dress with low neckline edged with self-fabric ruffles, matching short sleeves, hem of skirt and hem of drawers, sash in contrast colour at high waist level. Heelless cloth shoes with bar straps and blunt toes. [7] 2-year-old boy, *c.* 1810. Dress with off-the-shoulder neckline, ruched bodice trimmed with brass buttons, matching short sleeves, knee-length skirt with tucked detail. Short drawers with lace trim. Heelless cloth shoes with ribbon ties and blunt toes.

1812 – 1817

[1] 12-year-old boy, *c.* 1812. Single-breasted wool tailcoat with high collar, wide revers with M-notch and tight sleeves with sewn cuffs. Single-breasted cloth waistcoat with stand collar. Shirt worn with matching stock. Ankle-length wool pantaloons with fall fronts. Knitted silk stockings. Heelless leather shoes with ties above pointed toes. [2] 12-year-old boy, *c.* 1812. Double-breasted wool tailcoat with high collar, wide revers with M-notch, and tight sleeves with sewn cuffs and button trim. Collarless single-breasted waistcoat. Shirt worn with matching stock. Wool pantaloons tucked into heelless knee-length leather boots with shaped tops, tassel trim and blunt toes. [3] 8-year-old girl, *c.* 1817. Above-ankle-length wool and silk mixture dress with raised pattern, low neckline, ruched bodice and puff sleeves. Ankle-length drawers with lace trim. Knitted silk stockings. Heelless silk slippers with pointed toes. [4] 5-year-old girl, *c.* 1815. Wool outdoor dress with small collar above concealed opening, puff oversleeves with self-fabric petal-shaped epaulettes, long undersleeves with sewn cuffs, high waist-belt and mid-calf-length skirt with tucked hem detail, edges and detail piped in contrast colour. Drawers with lace trim. Straw bonnet with tall crown and fancy ribbon trim, bow tie under chin. Cloth gloves. Heelless cloth boots with side lacing and pointed toes. [5] 5-year-old boy, *c.* 1817. Cotton dress with low square neckline, ruched bodice, puff sleeves and knee-length skirt with tucked hem detail, matching ankle-length drawers. Straw hat with wide brim, tall crown and ribbon and bow trim. Heelless cloth boots with side lacing and pointed toes. [6] 3-year-old girl, *c.* 1816. Checked silk dress with low neckline, ruched bodice, puff sleeves and ankle-length skirt with tucked hem detail, matching full-length apron. Heelless silk shoes with ties over pointed toes. [7] 10-year-old girl, *c.* 1815. Fine wool outdoor dress with concealed opening under small contrast-colour collar, matching decorative tabs and cuffs on puff oversleeves, long undersleeves with sewn cuffs, high waist-belt, mid-calf-length skirt with tucked hem detail. Ankle-length cotton drawers with tucked detail above hems. Large straw hat with looped ribbon trim, bow tie under chin. Cloth gloves. Knitted silk stockings. Heelless leather shoes with side-laced fastenings above square toes.

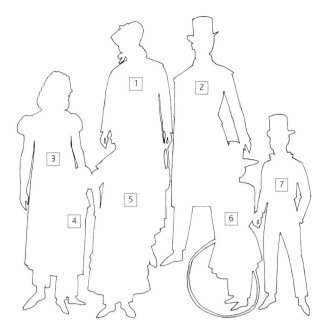

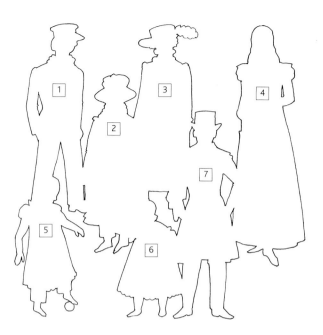

1818–1820

1 10-year-old girl, *c.* 1818. Mid-calf-length wool coat with small satin-edged lace-trimmed collar, matching shoulder-wide cape, edges of front button opening and cuffs of long sleeves. Straw hat with turned-down brim and shallow crown, fancy ribbon trim and bow tie under chin. Embroidered bag with long handles and tassel trim. Cloth gloves. Slippers with pointed toes. 2 12-year-old boy, *c.* 1820. Knee-length wool coat with small velvet collar, matching pocket flaps, buttons of single-breasted fastening and button trim on split cuffs of tight sleeves, shoulder cape, fitted body and full skirts. Cotton shirt with high collar and matching stock. Ankle-length wool trousers. Top hat with curled brim. Heelless cloth boots with side lacing and square toes. 3 9-year-old girl, *c.* 1820. Patterned cotton dress with inserted V-shaped pin-tucked panel with decorative button detail in ruched bodice under low neckline, matching puff sleeves and hem of mid-calf-length skirt. Ankle-length cotton drawers with lace trim. Knitted cotton stockings. Heelless cloth slippers with pointed toes. 4 3-year-old boy, *c.* 1820. Cotton dress with ruched bodice, low neckline with lace trim, matching short sleeves, tucked hems of knee-length skirt and ankle-length drawers. Knitted cotton stockings. Heelless cloth shoes with buttoned bar straps and pointed toes. 5 5-year-old girl, *c.* 1819. Fine wool coat with button fastening from under small stand collar to high waist, puff oversleeves, long undersleeves with frilled cuffs, matching shoulder cape and hem of knee-length skirts. Dress with tucked and pleated hem detail. Ankle-length cotton drawers with lace trim. Straw bonnet with frill-edged brim, ribbon and bow trim, bow tie under chin. Heelless cloth boots with side lacing and pointed toes. 6 4-year-old boy, *c.* 1820. Cotton dress with frill collar, ruched bodice with inserted bands of contrast-colour ribbon, matching cuffs of long sleeves, knee-length gathered skirt under low waist-belt, matching drawers. Straw hat with tall crown and wide brim. Knitted cotton stockings. Heelless cloth shoes with buttoned bar straps and square toes. 7 6-year-old boy, *c.* 1820. Double-breasted short wool jacket with M-notch collar and revers and tight sleeves with sewn cuffs and button trim. Cotton shirt with wide frill collar. Ankle-length wool trousers with fall fronts. Top hat with high crown and curled brim. Knitted cotton stockings. Heelless leather shoes with square toes.

1821–1822

1 6-year-old boy, *c.* 1822. Waist-length wool jacket with fitted bodice, concealed hook and bar fastening, three rows of decorative brass buttons, shaped hem with front point, long sleeves with sewn cuffs. Cotton shirt with frill collar. Wool trousers with fall fronts and stirrups under feet. Peaked cap. Leather shoes with low heels. 2 4-year-old girl, *c.* 1822. Fine wool dress, bodice decorated with diagonal tucks from centre front above high waist-belt, shoulder-wide collar with frilled edge, matching cuffs of long sleeves and scalloped trim above mid-calf-length hemline. Long cotton drawers with lace trim. Cloth hat with wide brim and gathered crown, ribbon biding and trim, bow tie under chin. Knitted silk stockings. Heelless cloth boots, laced from under ankle-level cuffs to above patent-leather pointed toecaps. 3 5-year-old girl, *c.* 1822. Short wool jacket with horizontal pin-tucked bodice, concealed hook and bar fastening, stand collar, long sleeves, fur epaulettes, matching edges and detail. Mid-calf-length dress with tucked detail above hemline. Ankle-length lace-trimmed cotton drawers. Straw hat with wide brim and tall crown, trimmed with embroidered ribbon and ostrich feather. Leather gloves. Cloth shoes with crossed ribbon straps and square toes. 4 10-year-old girl, *c.* 1822. Floral-embroidered silk party dress with wide neckline and narrow collar, ruched bodice above high waist-belt, puff sleeves with button trim, ankle-length skirt with single tuck above hemline. Beaded drawstring bag with long handles. Knitted silk stockings. Heelless silk satin slippers with crossed ribbon straps and square toes. 5 2-year-old boy, *c.* 1821. Cotton dress with low neckline, ruched bodice trimmed with buttons, puff sleeves and short skirt with decorative apron front, tucked hem, matching drawers. Knitted cotton stockings. Heelless cloth slippers with blunt toes. 6 1-year-old boy, *c.* 1821. Silk dress with ruched bodice, off-the-shoulder neckline with frilled edge, matching puff sleeves and hemline of short skirt. Two transparent silk underskirts with lace trim. Silk bonnet with frilled edge, ribbon rosette trim, bow tie under chin. Knitted cotton stockings. Heelless kid slippers with bow ties and blunt toes. 7 7-year-old boy, *c.* 1821. Wool tweed coat with fitted bodice, centre-front hook and bar fastening, three rows of decorative brass buttons, matching trim on sewn cuffs of long sleeves, collar above shoulder cape, buckled belt, knee-length skirts. Cotton shirt with high collar and silk cravat. Wool trousers with stirrups under feet. Silk top hat. Leather gloves. Cloth ankle boots with low heels and square patent-leather toecaps.

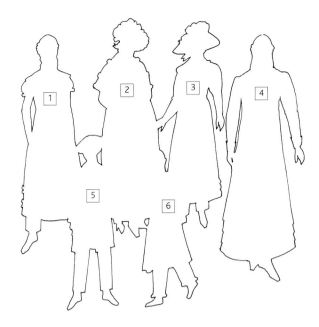

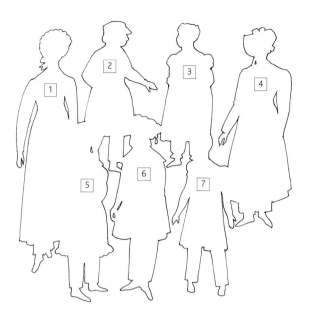

1823 – 1825

1 8-year-old girl, *c.* 1825. Silk party dress with wide neckline edged with frill, puff sleeves with rosette trim, tight bodice with braid-trimmed panel seams, matching edges of high waist-belt and trimming on ankle-length skirt, hemline also decorated with rosettes and frills. Cotton drawers with tucked hem detail. Hair dressed with flowers. Pearl necklace. Cotton gloves. Knitted silk stockings. Heelless silk slippers with flower trim above square toes. 2 9-year-old girl, *c.* 1823. Mid-calf-length cashmere coat with long sleeves, ribbon tie under marabou-trimmed collar, matching two-tier cape, front edges, hem and small hand muff. Dress with frills at neck and hem. Cloth bonnet with tall crown trimmed with ostrich feather and embroidered ribbon, matching tie under chin and brim edge. Heelless cloth boots with square patent-leather toecaps. 3 8-year-old girl, *c.* 1825. Ankle-length fine wool outdoor dress with frill-edged collar, shoulder-wide broderie-anglaise-trimmed yoke, matching cuffs on leg-of-mutton sleeves, tight bodice with vertical tucks above high-waisted embroidered belt, skirt hem trimmed with matching embroidery, frills and broderie anglaise. Ankle-length cotton drawers. Cloth hat with gathered crown and wide brim, ribbon trim, bow tie under chin. Knitted silk stockings. Heelless cloth slippers with crossed ribbon straps and square toes. 4 10-year-old girl, *c.* 1824. Ankle-length striped cotton dress with fitted bodice above high-waisted self-fabric buckled belt, broderie-anglaise collar, matching cuffs on leg-of-mutton sleeves and trim between tucks above hem. Knitted cotton stockings. Heelless cloth slippers with crossed ribbon ties and square toes. 5 6-year-old boy, *c.* 1825. Knee-length striped cotton coat-dress with single-breasted button fastening, long sleeves with stitched cuffs, self-fabric buckled belt and matching trousers. Cotton shirt with large frill-edged collar, worn with ribbon bow. Brimless beret with bow trim on one side. Knitted cotton stockings. Heelless leather shoes with buckle trim and square toes. 6 4-year-old boy, *c.* 1823. Knee-length cotton coat-dress with frills around neckline and sleeve hems, concealed hook and bar fastening, brass button trim, self-fabric buckled belt, long sleeves with braid-trimmed sewn cuffs, matching edges and detail and decoration on hem of skirts. Ankle-length trousers in matching fabric and trim. Knitted cotton stockings. Heelless cloth slippers with square toes.

1826 – 1827

1 12-year-old girl, *c.* 1827. Mid-calf-length spotted cotton voile dress with contrast-colour high waist-belt, matching buttoned cuffs on full-length leg-of-mutton sleeves, bindings and trim on low neckline and piping on ruched bodice, ruched detail repeated under neckline. Ankle-length cotton drawers with lace trim. Bonnet with ruched inner brim, ostrich feather trim, ribbon bow tied under chin. Knitted silk stockings. Heelless cloth slippers with crossed ribbon straps and square toes. 2 4-year-old boy, *c.* 1826. Knee-length striped cotton dress with single-breasted button fastening from under lace collar to hem, matching lace cuffs on long sleeves, fitted bodice, full skirt and buttoned waist-belt. Checked silk scarf tied at front. Ankle-length cotton drawers with lace trim. Cloth cap with cord trim and stiffened peak. Knitted cotton stockings. Heelless cloth slippers. 3 4-year-old girl, *c.* 1827. Mid-calf-length silk dress with low neckline, puff sleeves and split oversleeves, ruched bodice above high waist-belt and gathered skirt. Cotton drawers gathered into ankle-level band. Knitted silk stockings. Heelless cloth slippers. 4 7-year-old girl, *c.* 1826. Mid-calf-length wool coat with single-breasted fastening from under lace-trimmed collar to hem, high waist-belt with buckle, all edges bound with velvet, matching cuffs of leg-of-mutton sleeves and covered buttons. Skirt with tucked hem detail. Ankle-length cotton drawers. Dyed straw bonnet with satin ribbon binding and trim. Cloth gloves. Knitted silk stockings. Heelless slippers with bow trim and square toes. 5 5-year-old girl, *c.* 1826. Knee-length fine cotton dress with two shoulder-wide collars trimmed with ribbon and edged with frills, matching hem of gathered skirt, leg-of-mutton sleeves with cuffs, contrast-colour high waist-belt and bow tie. Ankle-length lace-trimmed cotton drawers. Straw hat with ribbon binding and trim. Knitted cotton stockings. Heelless cloth slippers with crossed straps and square toes. 6 5-year-old boy, *c.* 1826. Knee-length wool coat with double-breasted brass button fastening to waist, trim on lace-edged sewn cuffs of leg-of-mutton sleeves matching lace trim on shoulder-wide collar. Silk neck scarf. Ankle-length striped wool trousers. Velvet beret. Cloth gloves. Knitted cotton stockings. Heelless leather shoes with buckle trim and square toes. 7 3-year-old boy, *c.* 1826. Knee-length cotton dress split at centre front, high waist, puff sleeves, ruched bodice and low frill-edged neckline, lace-trimmed edges and detail. Ankle-length lace-trimmed cotton drawers. Knitted cotton stockings. Heelless cloth slippers with bar straps and blunt toes.

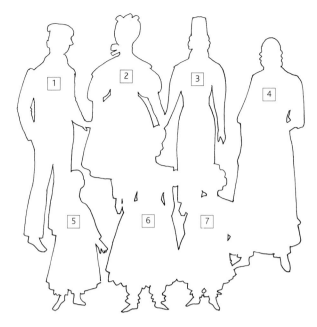

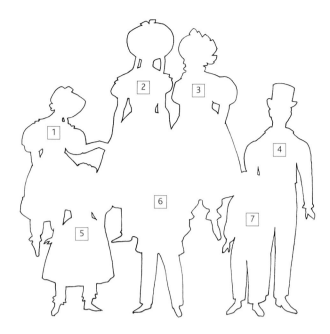

1828 – 1830

1 9-year-old boy, *c.* 1830. Short single-breasted wool jacket with long shawl collar and long sleeves with shaped sewn cuffs. Single-breasted wool waistcoat with shawl collar. Cotton shirt with stand collar and pin-tucked front. Silk neck scarf. Wool trousers with straight legs and fall fronts. Cloth cap, high crown with gathered top, small peak and leather chin strap. Knitted cotton stockings. Heelless leather slippers with bow trim above square toes. 2 6-year-old girl, *c.* 1829. Velvet dress with large puff sleeves attached to tight sleeves with buttoned trim, high waist-belt with buckle, full skirt with fringe trimming above hem, matching hem of single-breasted shoulder cape, pleated cotton ruffle at neck. Lace-trimmed cotton drawers. Bonnet with pleated inner brim, looped embroidered ribbon trim and ties under chin. Cloth gloves. Knitted silk stockings. Heelless leather slippers with square toes. 3 6-year-old boy, *c.* 1830. Single-breasted wool top with shawl collar and leg-of-mutton sleeves with buttoned cuffs, top worn tucked into deep waistband of ankle-length trousers, brass button fastenings and trim. Collarless cotton shirt. Stiffened cloth cap with tall ribbon-trimmed crown and narrow peak. Knitted cotton stockings. Heelless leather slippers with buttoned bar straps and square toes. 4 12-year-old girl, *c.* 1828. Ankle-length embroidered muslin dress, low neckline with pleated edge, narrow yoke, ruched bodice, elbow-length gathered sleeves, tight lower sleeves banded with lace above shaped cuffs, apron-effect panels attached to high waistband over ankle-length skirt with frill at knee level. Lace-trimmed cotton drawers. Large straw hat with looped ribbon trim and long ties. Knitted cotton stockings. Heelless silk slippers with bow trim and pointed toes. 5 2-year-old girl, *c.* 1830. Patterned cotton dress, low neckline with pleated edge, matching hems of three-quarter-length sleeves, full skirt gathered from high waist, decorative tucks above hem. Lace-trimmed cotton drawers. Heelless cloth ankle boots with patent-leather trim and square toecaps. 6 7-year-old girl, *c.* 1830. Spotted cotton dress with low lace-trimmed neckline, matching hems of puff sleeves and wide band below tucked hemline. Striped cotton pinafore with wide shoulder straps gathered into wide waistband and full skirt with small patch pockets. Lace-trimmed cotton drawers gathered into ankle-level band. Bonnet with draped crown and back frill, ribbon binding and ties. Heelless cloth ankle boots with square leather toecaps trimmed with buttons. 7 2-year-old girl, *c.* 1830. Cotton dress with puff sleeves, low lace-trimmed neckline, matching decoration on bodice, full skirt gathered from under high waistband, frilled hemline. Lace-trimmed cotton drawers gathered into ankle-level band. Knitted cotton stockings. Heelless leather slippers with ribbon ties and square toes.

1831 – 1833

1 5-year-old girl, *c.* 1831. Silk taffeta dress with low lace-edged neckline, pin-tucked bodice, large puff sleeves above tight lower sleeves with turned-back cuffs, knee-length skirt gathered from under buckled high waist-belt, self-fabric pleated frill from shoulder to above hem front and back on both sides. Cotton drawers gathered at ankle level. Straw bonnet with embroidered ribbon trim and ties. Knitted silk stockings. Heelless silk slippers with square toes. 2 8-year-old girl, *c.* 1833. Spotted voile dress with low neckline, pleated cross-over bodice and in-fill, double frill above puff sleeves, mid-calf-length skirt with frilled hemline, box-pleats from under wide waistband. Ankle-length lace-trimmed drawers. Straw hat with wide brim and silk ribbon trim and ties. Knitted cotton stockings. Heelless silk slippers with square toes. 3 7-year-old girl, *c.* 1831. Wool coat with woven patterned stripe, mid-calf-length skirt gathered under wide waistband, two rows of fur trim above hem, matching cuffs on tight sleeves, centre-front bodice above concealed fastening, neckline and tiny hand muff. Cotton drawers gathered at ankle level. Silk bonnet with pleated inner brim, tall crown, embroidered ribbon trim and ties under chin. Knitted silk stockings. Heelless silk slippers with cross-over ribbon straps and square toes. 4 8-year-old boy, *c.* 1832. Single-breasted wool tailcoat with shawl collar and leg-of-mutton sleeves. Single-breasted silk waistcoat with notched shawl collar and pointed front. Cotton shirt with pleated collar and cuffs. Silk neck tie. Straight-cut wool trousers with fall fronts. Top hat with curled brim. Heelless cloth ankle boots with low heels and square patent-leather toecaps. 5 5-year-old girl, *c.* 1832. Striped silk top with low lace-edged neckline, matching pointed scalloped hem and sewn cuffs of tight lower sleeves under large puff sleeves. Plain contrast-colour gathered skirt and waist-belt. Ankle-length lace-trimmed cotton drawers. Knitted silk stockings. Heelless silk slippers with square toes. 6 4-year-old boy, *c.* 1831. Double-breasted flecked wool jacket, cut to be worn open, brass buttons, matching trim on sewn cuffs of long sleeves. Single-breasted collarless silk waistcoat with point at front. Cotton shirt with frill-edged collar. Ankle-length trousers in flecked wool. Knitted silk stockings. Heelless leather slippers with square toes. 7 2-year-old boy, *c.* 1832. Short velvet top, ruched front bodice with button fastening, matching buttoned cuffs on leg-of-mutton sleeves, worn over cotton shirt with pleated collar and cuffs. Top buttoned to ankle-length silk trousers. Knitted silk stockings. Heelless silk slippers with square toes.

Infants' Frocks 1800–1850

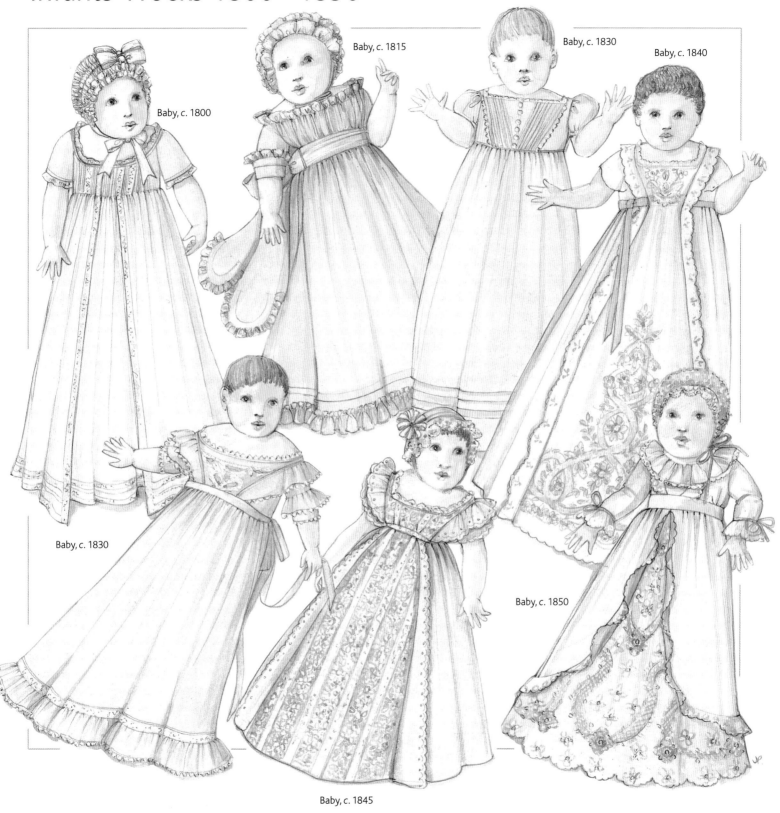

Baby, c. 1800

Baby, c. 1815

Baby, c. 1830

Baby, c. 1840

Baby, c. 1830

Baby, c. 1845

Baby, c. 1850

1834–1835

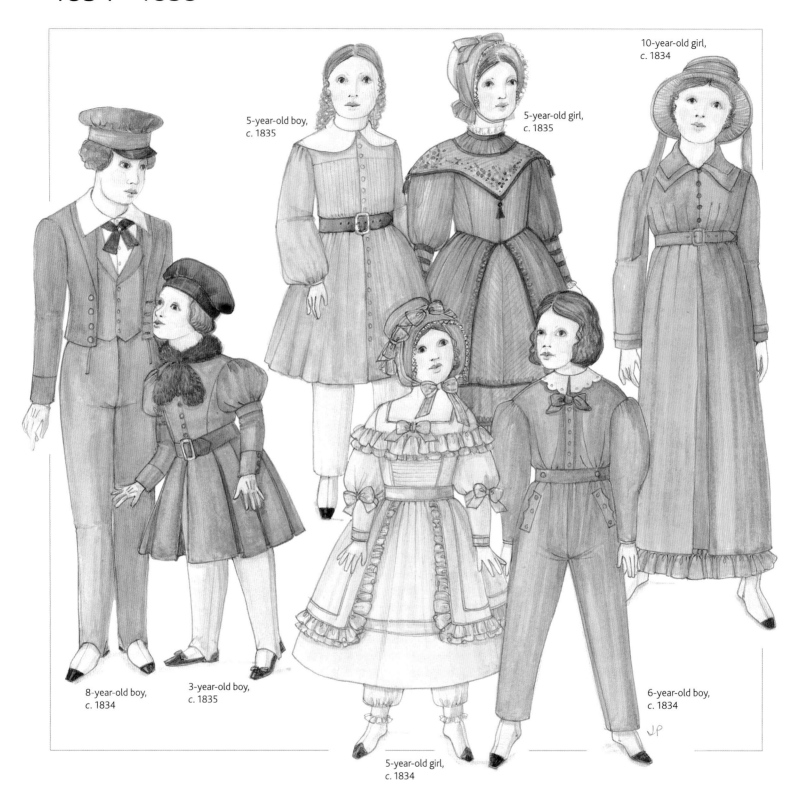

5-year-old boy,
c. 1835

10-year-old girl,
c. 1834

5-year-old girl,
c. 1835

8-year-old boy,
c. 1834

3-year-old boy,
c. 1835

6-year-old boy,
c. 1834

5-year-old girl,
c. 1834

1836 – 1838

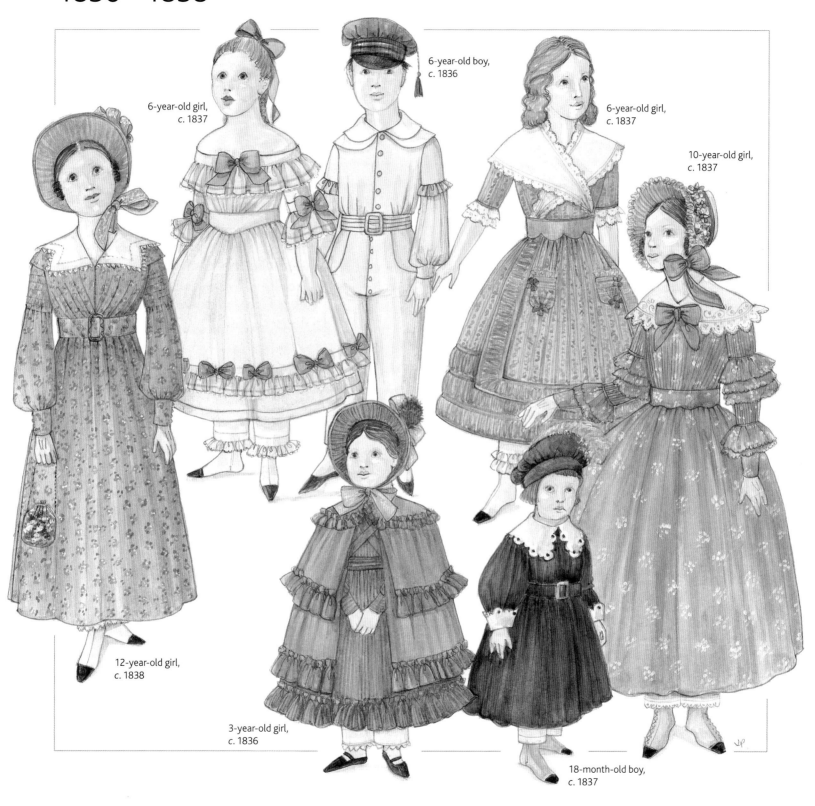

6-year-old girl,
c. 1837

6-year-old boy,
c. 1836

6-year-old girl,
c. 1837

10-year-old girl,
c. 1837

12-year-old girl,
c. 1838

3-year-old girl,
c. 1836

18-month-old boy,
c. 1837

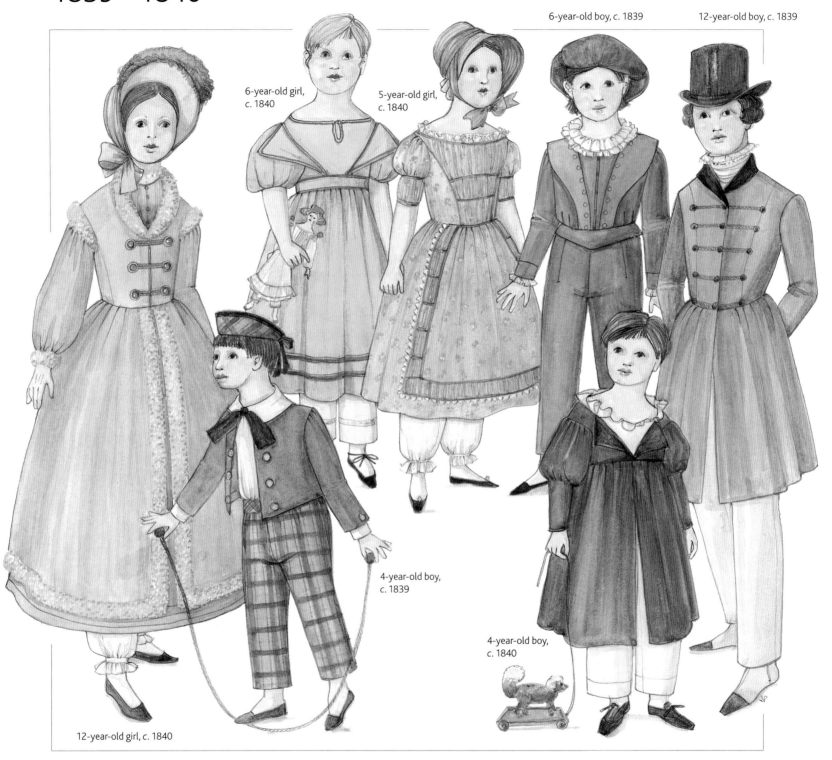

6-year-old boy, *c.* 1839

12-year-old boy, *c.* 1839

6-year-old girl,
c. 1840

5-year-old girl,
c. 1840

4-year-old boy,
c. 1839

4-year-old boy,
c. 1840

12-year-old girl, *c.* 1840

1841–1842

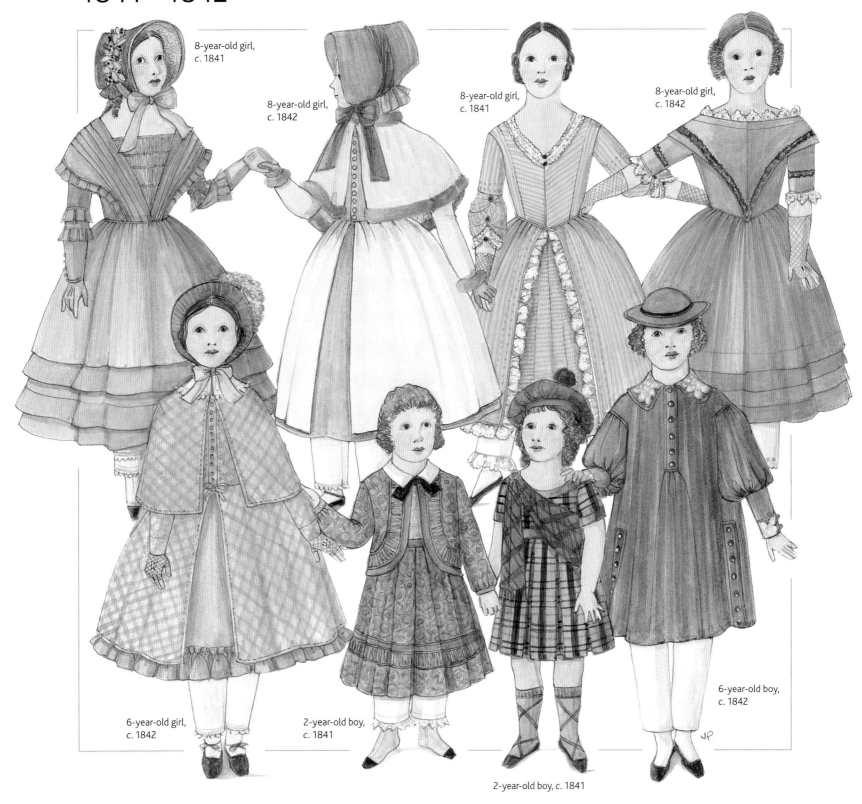

8-year-old girl, *c.* 1841

8-year-old girl, *c.* 1842

8-year-old girl, *c.* 1841

8-year-old girl, *c.* 1842

6-year-old girl, *c.* 1842

2-year-old boy, *c.* 1841

2-year-old boy, *c.* 1841

6-year-old boy, *c.* 1842

1843–1844

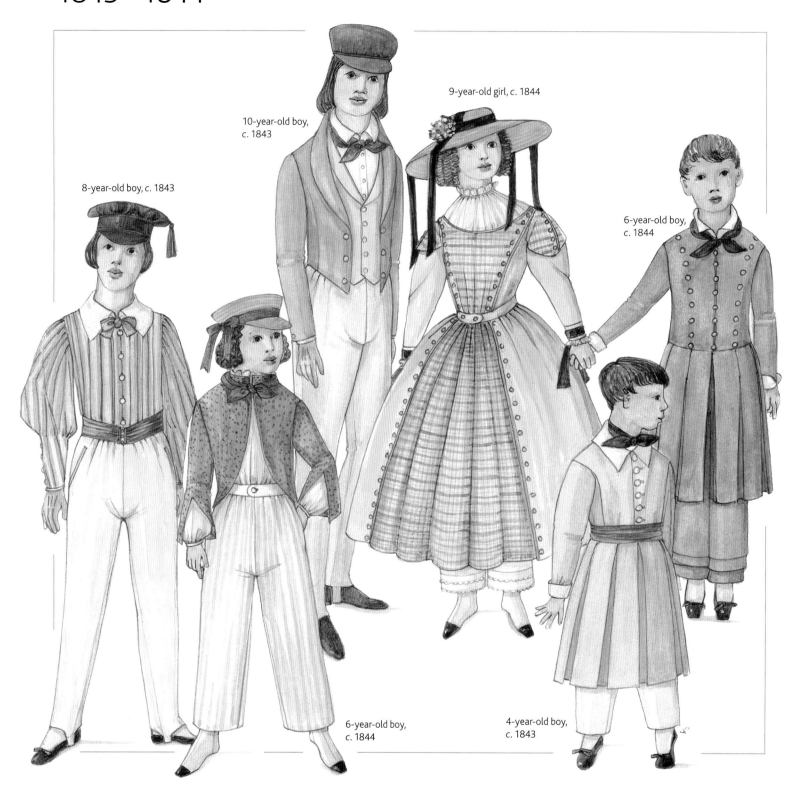

8-year-old boy, *c.* 1843

10-year-old boy,
c. 1843

9-year-old girl, *c.* 1844

6-year-old boy,
c. 1844

6-year-old boy,
c. 1844

4-year-old boy,
c. 1843

1845–1846

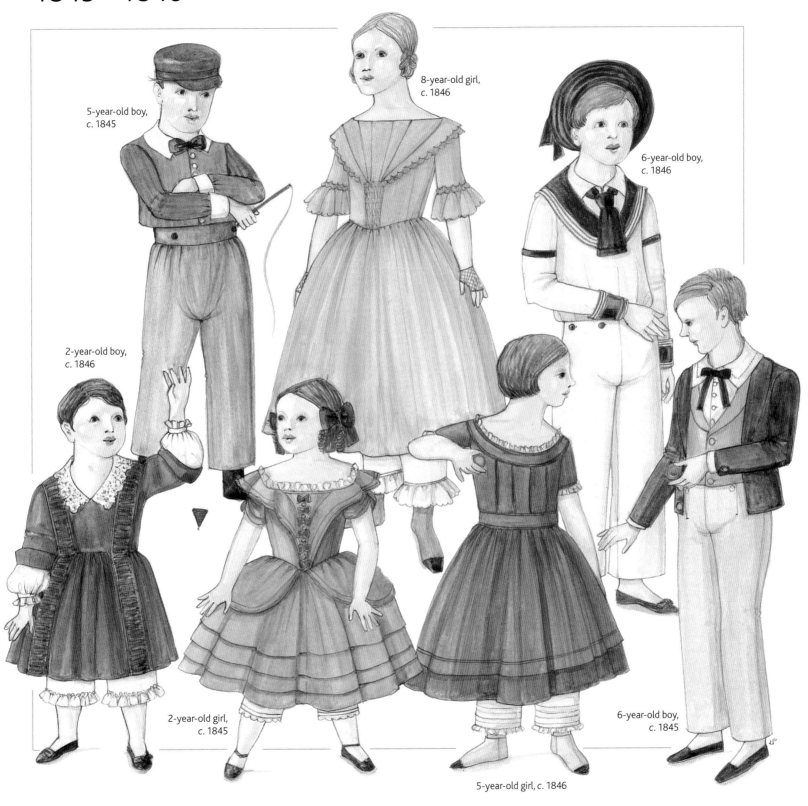

5-year-old boy, *c.* 1845

8-year-old girl, *c.* 1846

6-year-old boy, *c.* 1846

2-year-old boy, *c.* 1846

2-year-old girl, *c.* 1845

5-year-old girl, *c.* 1846

6-year-old boy, *c.* 1845

1847–1849

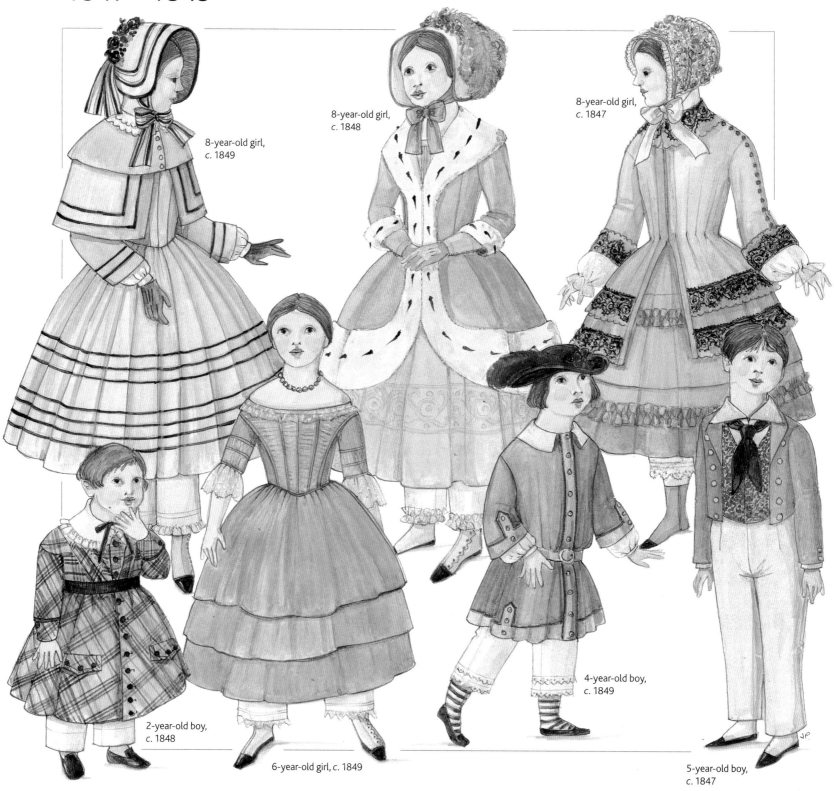

8-year-old girl, c. 1849

8-year-old girl, c. 1848

8-year-old girl, c. 1847

2-year-old boy, c. 1848

6-year-old girl, c. 1849

4-year-old boy, c. 1849

5-year-old boy, c. 1847

1850–1851

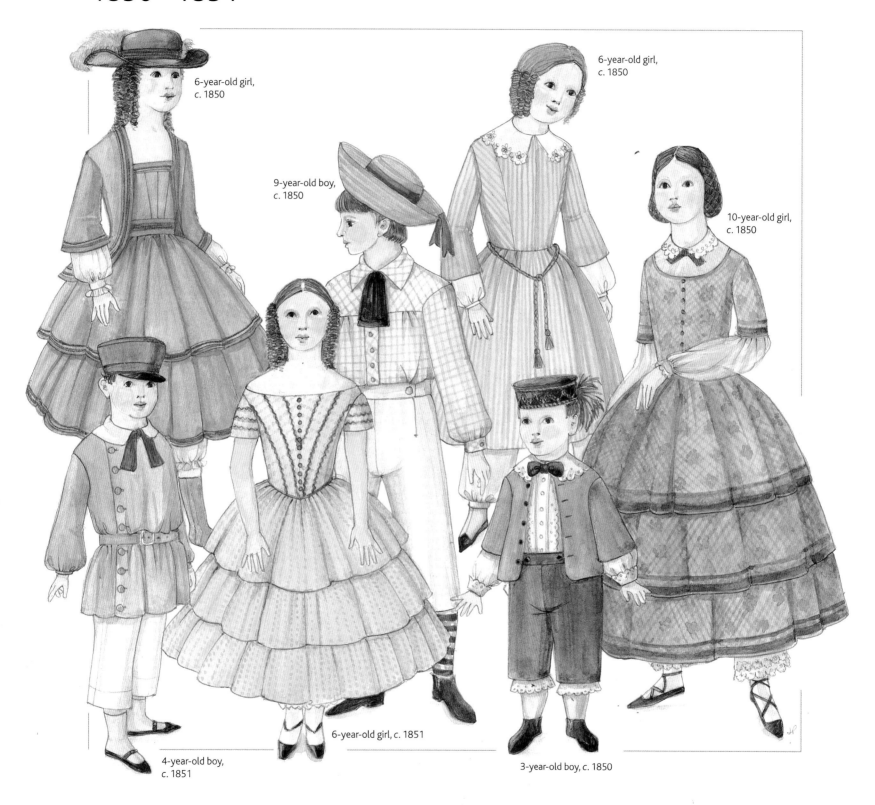

6-year-old girl, c. 1850

9-year-old boy, c. 1850

6-year-old girl, c. 1850

10-year-old girl, c. 1850

4-year-old boy, c. 1851

6-year-old girl, c. 1851

3-year-old boy, c. 1850

1852–1854

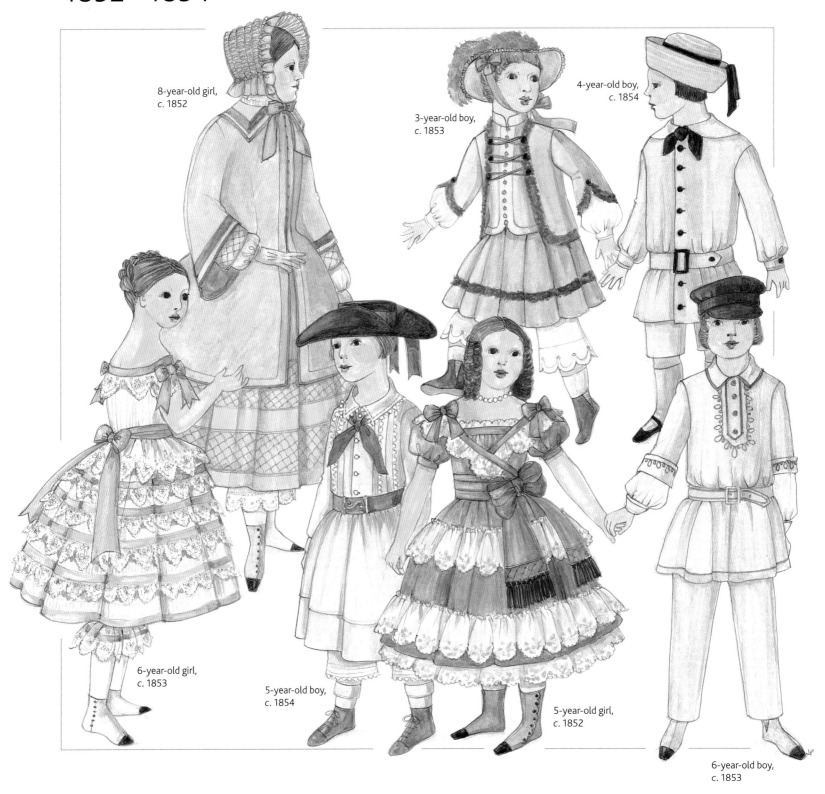

8-year-old girl,
c. 1852

3-year-old boy,
c. 1853

4-year-old boy,
c. 1854

6-year-old girl,
c. 1853

5-year-old boy,
c. 1854

5-year-old girl,
c. 1852

6-year-old boy,
c. 1853

1855–1856

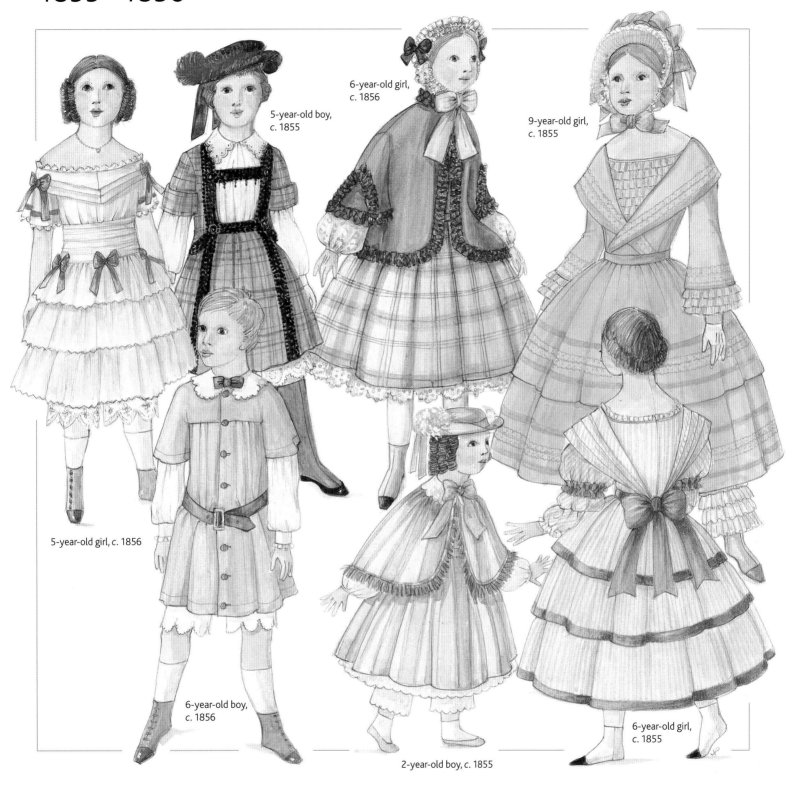

5-year-old boy,
c. 1855

6-year-old girl,
c. 1856

9-year-old girl,
c. 1855

5-year-old girl, c. 1856

6-year-old boy,
c. 1856

2-year-old boy, c. 1855

6-year-old girl,
c. 1855

1857–1858

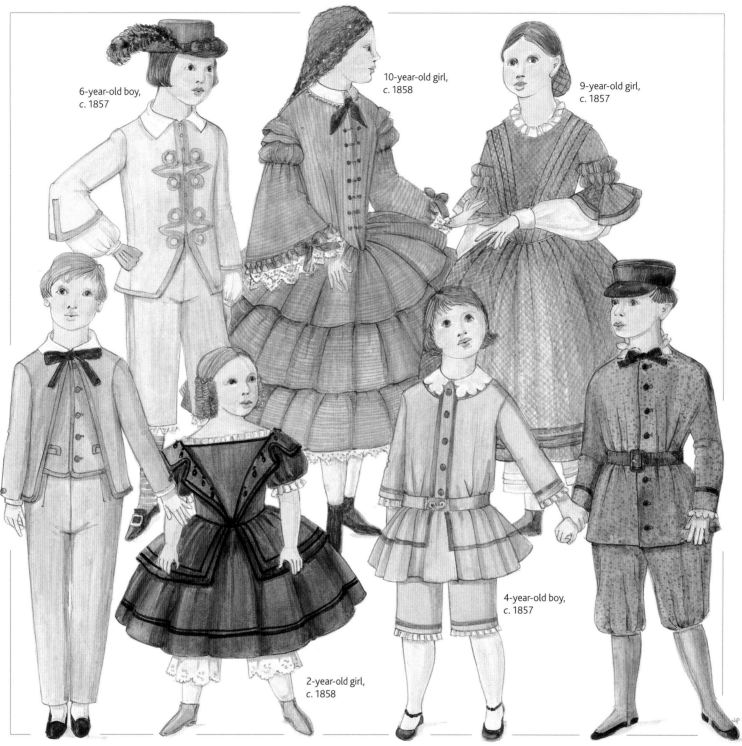

6-year-old boy, c. 1857

10-year-old girl, c. 1858

9-year-old girl, c. 1857

2-year-old girl, c. 1858

4-year-old boy, c. 1857

5-year-old boy, c. 1857

5-year-old boy, c. 1858

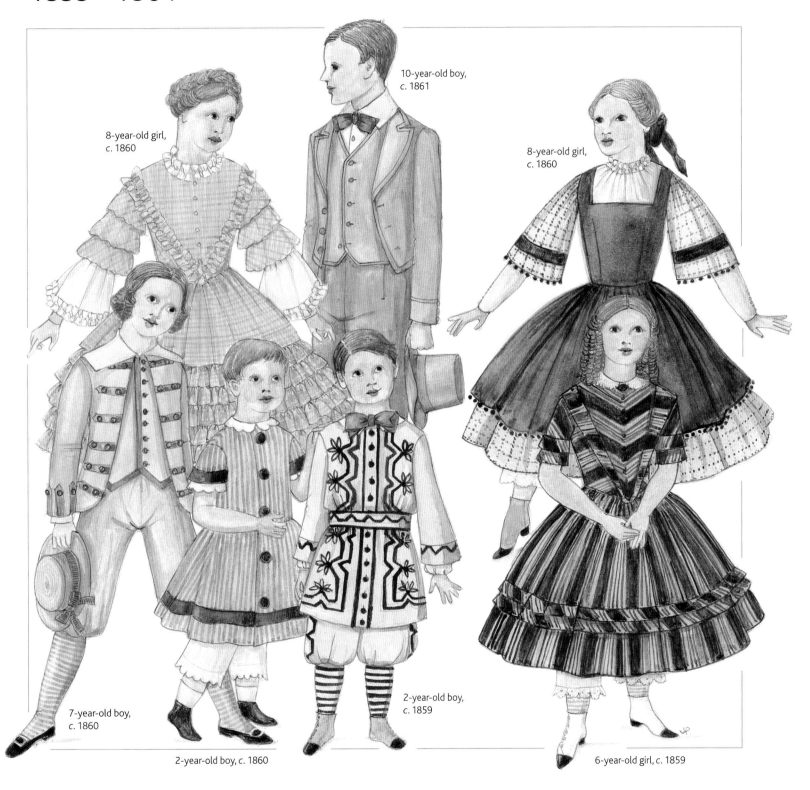

8-year-old girl,
c. 1860

10-year-old boy,
c. 1861

8-year-old girl,
c. 1860

7-year-old boy,
c. 1860

2-year-old boy, *c.* 1860

2-year-old boy,
c. 1859

6-year-old girl, *c.* 1859

1862–1863

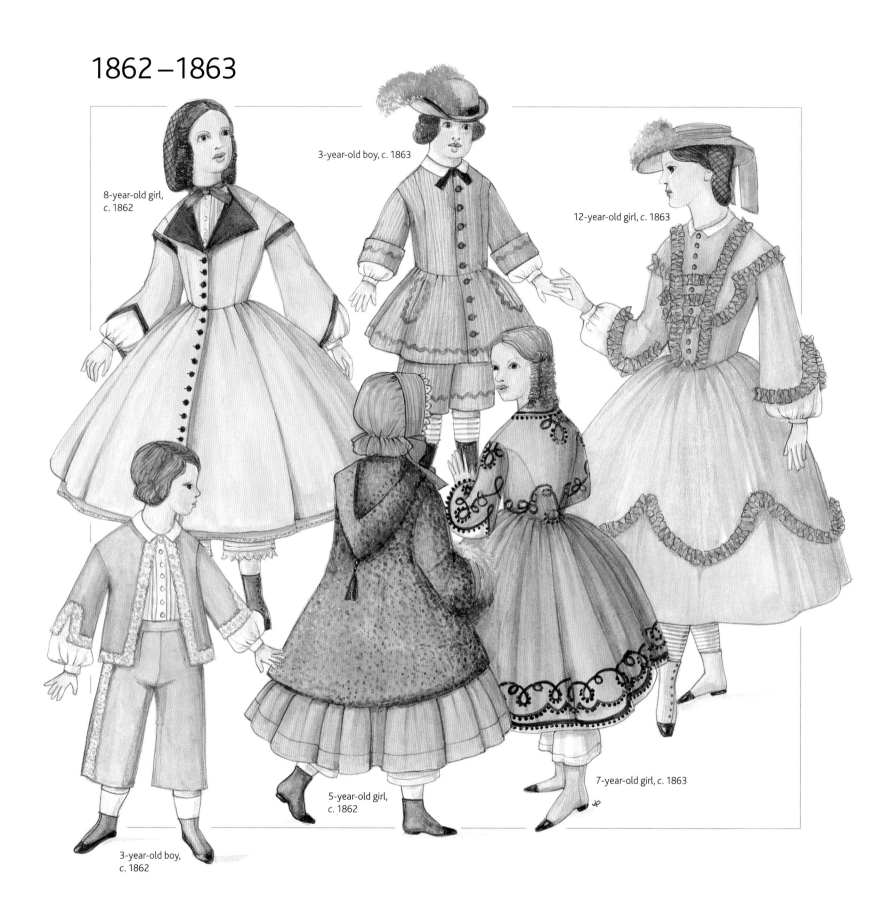

8-year-old girl, c. 1862

3-year-old boy, c. 1863

12-year-old girl, c. 1863

3-year-old boy, c. 1862

5-year-old girl, c. 1862

7-year-old girl, c. 1863

1864–1866

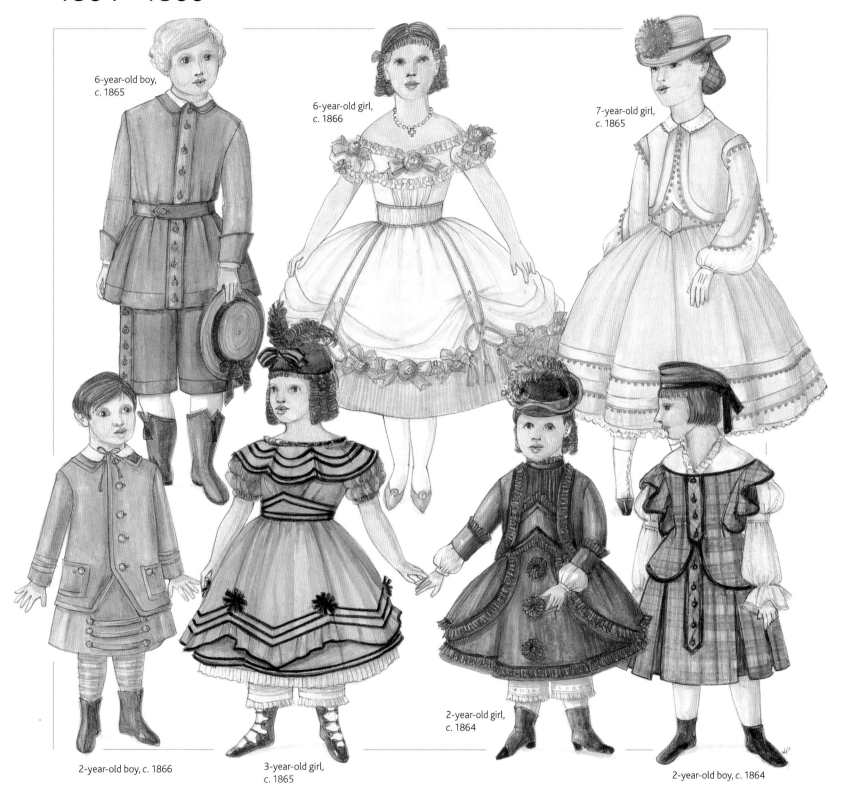

6-year-old boy,
c. 1865

6-year-old girl,
c. 1866

7-year-old girl,
c. 1865

2-year-old boy, c. 1866

3-year-old girl,
c. 1865

2-year-old girl,
c. 1864

2-year-old boy, c. 1864

Hats 1800 –1866

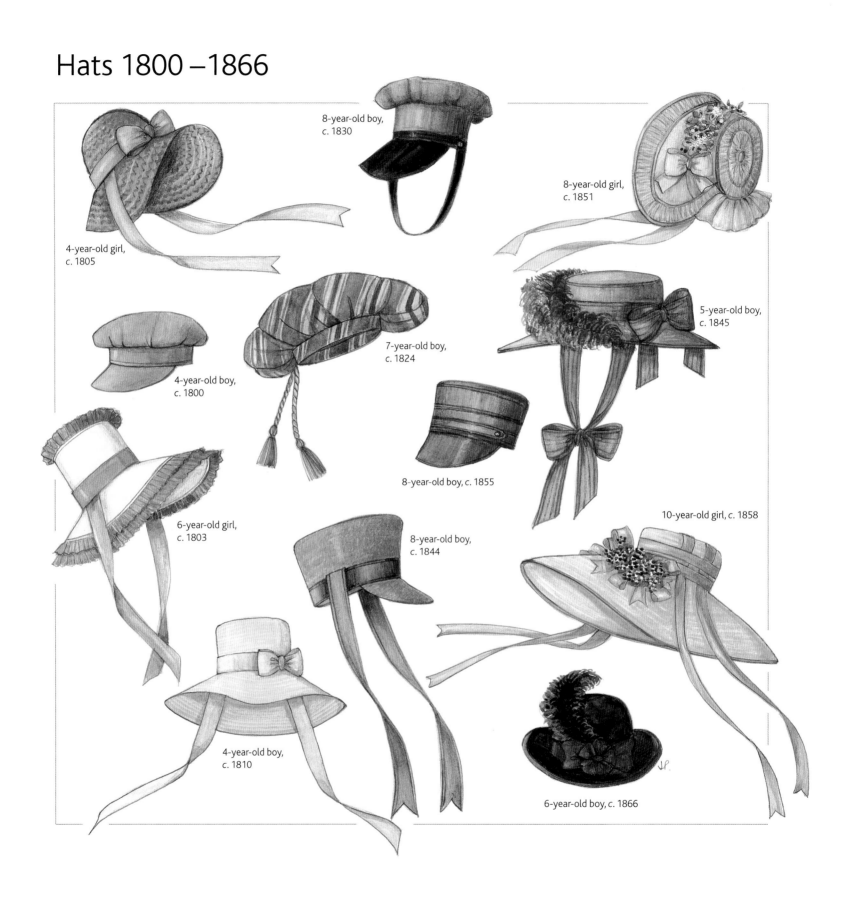

8-year-old boy,
c. 1830

8-year-old girl,
c. 1851

4-year-old girl,
c. 1805

5-year-old boy,
c. 1845

7-year-old boy,
c. 1824

4-year-old boy,
c. 1800

8-year-old boy, *c.* 1855

10-year-old girl, *c.* 1858

6-year-old girl,
c. 1803

8-year-old boy,
c. 1844

4-year-old boy,
c. 1810

6-year-old boy, *c.* 1866

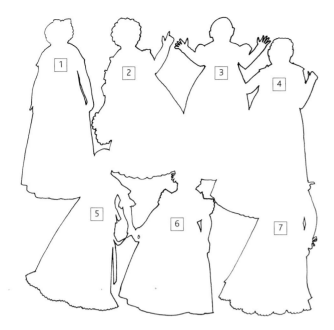

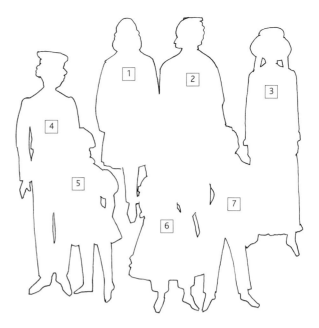

Infants' Frocks 1800 – 1850

1 Baby, *c.* 1800. Cotton muslin frock with low round neckline edged with lace, matching hems of short inset sleeves, trim between pin tucks on front of short bodice and edges and hems of over- and underskirts. Frilled and ruched cotton muslin bonnet with double satin ribbon bow trim, matching ties under chin. 2 Baby, *c.* 1815. Fine cotton frock with short ruched bodice and low frill-edged off-the-shoulder neckline, matching trim on cuffs of three-quarter-length inset sleeves, curved ends of wide waist-sash and on hemline of full skirt under pin-tucked detail. Deep frilled bonnet with ties under chin. 3 Baby, *c.* 1830. Cotton frock with low lace-edged square neckline, matching trim on each side of diagonal pin tucks on button-trimmed short bodice, short inset puff sleeves, long skirt with pin-tucked detail above hemline. 4 Baby, *c.* 1840. Cotton muslin frock with low lace-edged square neckline, short embroidered bodice above narrow silk ribbon belt tied into bow on one side, short inset sleeves, embroidered scallop-edged pleats from shoulders to hemline, richly embroidered skirt. 5 Baby, *c.* 1830. Cotton muslin frock with short lace-trimmed embroidered bodice at back and wide lace-edged off-the-shoulder neckline, matching hems of three-quarter-length inset sleeves with frill detail, epaulettes and hemline of full skirt. 6 Baby, *c.* 1845. Silk frock with low lace-edged round neckline, two-tier frilled epaulettes with scalloped edges, matching pleats on each side of full overskirt, underskirt embroidered and lace-trimmed to match short bodice. Silk bonnet with frilled lace edges, silk ribbon rosette trim on one side, matching ribbon ties under chin. 7 Baby, *c.* 1850. Fine silk frock, round neckline frilled with self-fabric and edged in fine lace, bias-cut scallop-edged waterfall frill from each shoulder of short bodice to hem of split overskirt, matching gathered frill on hems of long inset sleeves with ribbon trim, richly embroidered underskirt with scalloped hemline. Swansdown bonnet with lace undercap and ribbon ties under chin.

1834 – 1835

1 5-year-old boy, *c.* 1835. Single-breasted knee-length cotton coat with pin-tucked bodice, full-length gathered sleeves and shoulder-wide collar, worn with buckled leather waist-belt. Ankle-length cotton trousers. Heelless cloth ankle boots with leather soles and square toecaps. 2 5-year-old girl, *c.* 1835. Striped silk dress with tight bodice, high round neckline with frilled edge, repeated on hems of full-length sleeves, puffed to elbow level with bands of velvet trim to wrist, matching bindings on tassel-trimmed shoulder-wide embroidered collar, full skirt with braid decoration worn over stiffened petticoats. Straw bonnet with lace-edged brim and ribbon trimmings. 3 10-year-old girl, *c.* 1834. Single-breasted heavy cotton coat with ankle-length skirts, high waist-belt, large collar and full-length sleeves with decorative straps at wrist level. Ankle-length cotton dress with frilled hemline and large collar. Silk bonnet with ruched inner brim, contrast-colour band, bindings and ties. Heelless cloth ankle boots with leather soles and square toecaps. 4 8-year-old boy, *c.* 1834. Single-breasted short wool jacket with shawl collar and long sleeves with stitched cuffs, trousers in matching fabric with fall fronts, narrow legs and stirrups under instep. Single-breasted wool waistcoat with shawl collar. Cotton shirt with large pointed Peter Pan collar, worn with silk ribbon tie. Wool cap with gathered crown and leather peak. Short cotton gloves. Cloth ankle boots with leather soles, heels and square toecaps. 5 3-year-old boy, *c.* 1835. Single-breasted knee-length wool coat, long sleeves with stitched cuffs, button trim and puffed oversleeves, self-fabric buckled waist-belt above box-pleated skirts, worn with fur scarf and leather gloves. Wool trousers with stirrups under instep. Brimless velvet cap. Knitted silk stockings. Heelless leather shoes with bow trim and square toes. 6 5-year-old girl, *c.* 1834. Mid-calf-length silk dress, tight bodice with panel of horizontal pin tucks, full-length sleeves puffed to elbow level and trimmed with self-fabric bow, repeated under low square neckline, off-the-shoulder double row of self-fabric frills, matching trim on edges and hem of open overskirt, full skirt worn over stiffened underskirts. Straw bonnet with lace-edged brim, embroidered ribbon trim and ties. Full-length drawers gathered into frilled band at ankle level. Heelless cloth ankle boots with leather soles and square toecaps. 7 6-year-old boy, *c.* 1834. Single-breasted cotton blouse with leg-of-mutton sleeves, lace collar with coloured bow tie attached below, blouse buttoned onto waistband of ankle-length trousers in matching fabric with two side hip pockets with button trim. Heelless cloth boots with leather soles and square toecaps.

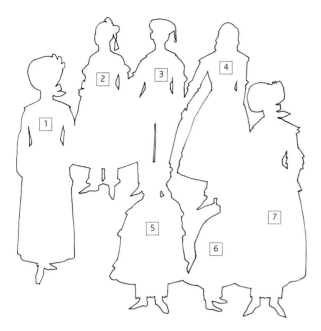

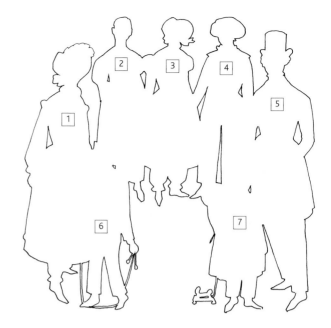

1836–1838

1 12-year-old girl, *c.* 1838. Printed cotton dress with fitted bodice, high waist emphasized by embroidered belt with steel buckle, V-shaped neckline with large lace-edged plain cotton collar, long sleeves gathered into buttoned cuffs, ruched upper sleeves under tiny caps, full ankle-length skirt. Bonnet with ruched inner brim, embroidered ribbon trim and ties under chin. Cloth gloves. Embroidered bag with long cord handle. Heelless cloth boots with leather soles and square toecaps. 2 6-year-old girl, *c.* 1837. Silk dress with fitted bodice, off-the-shoulder neckline edged with wide frill and trimmed with contrast-colour bow, matching hems of elbow-length sleeves and detail around hemline of full skirt. Ankle-length drawers with frilled hems. Hair ribbon with long ends. Heelless cloth boots with leather soles and square toecaps. 3 6-year-old boy, *c.* 1836. Single-breasted cotton blouse with long sleeves gathered into buttoned cuffs, inserted self-fabric gathered frill at elbow level, shoulder-wide two-tier contrast-colour collar. Ankle-length trousers under wide self-fabric belt, front button fastening, large hip-level pockets. Cap with gathered crown, wide band, leather peak, cord and tassel trim. Leather pumps with pointed toes. 4 6-year-old girl, *c.* 1837. Patterned cotton dress with large embroidered plain cotton collar crossed over fitted bodice, matching frills on hems of three-quarter-length sleeves, full skirt with rows of ruched detail above hemline, repeated on edges of decorative pinafore with two patch pockets, bindings, edges, detail and scalloped waistband in contrast colour. Ankle-length drawers with double frilled hems. Heelless cloth boots with leather soles and square toecaps. 5 3-year-old girl, *c.* 1836. Two-tier velvet cape fastened with crossed straps at front, shoulder-wide collar with frilled edge, matching hemlines on both tiers. Striped silk dress with high waist-belt, long sleeves gathered into cuffs, frilled hemline. Ankle-length drawers with lace trim. Large bonnet with ruched inner brim, feather and looped ribbon trim, matching ties under chin. Knitted silk stockings. Heelless cloth slippers with bar straps and pointed toes. 6 18-month-old boy, *c.* 1837. Knee-length velvet dress, high waist-belt with steel buckle, shoulder-wide embroidered collar, matching cuffs on full gathered sleeves. Ankle-length cotton drawers. Brimless velvet cap with gathered crown and feather trim. Heelless cloth boots with leather soles and toecaps. 7 10-year-old girl, *c.* 1837. Printed cotton dress with fitted pin-tucked bodice, matching sleeves between scalloped frills, shoulder-wide lace-edged and embroidered collar with bow trim, scalloped waistband, full skirt worn over stiffened petticoats. Ankle-length drawers with lace trim. Bonnet with ruched inner brim, crown decorated with silk flowers and ribbons, matching ties under chin. Cotton gloves. Heelless cloth boots with leather soles and square toecaps.

1839–1840

1 12-year-old girl, *c.* 1840. Single-breasted wool coat with fastening of double-breasted set buttons and braid trim, fitted bodice with fur collar, matching epaulettes and cuffs on long gathered sleeves and trim on edges and hems of full skirts. Cotton dress with lace-trimmed high round neckline and full skirt. Cotton drawers gathered into band at ankle level. Bonnet trimmed with ostrich feather, ribbon band and ties under chin. Cloth gloves. Knitted silk stockings. Heelless cloth slippers with leather soles and square toes. 2 6-year-old girl, *c.* 1840. Cotton dress, fitted bodice with wide neckline and keyhole opening at front, mock revers set into each side-bodice partly covering large puff sleeves, inset waistband and full skirt, contrast-colour piping, edges and trim. Ankle-length cotton drawers with inserted lace above hem. Knitted cotton stockings. Heelless leather shoes with ribbon ties and square toes. 3 5-year-old girl, *c.* 1840. Printed cotton dress, fitted bodice with wide frill-edged neckline, ruched detail between contrast-colour piping on front, matching cuffs under puff sleeves and border of decorative lace-trimmed apron worn over full skirt. Cotton drawers gathered at ankle level. Straw bonnet trimmed with ribbon, matching bow tie under chin. Knitted cotton stockings. Heelless cloth slippers with leather soles, bobble trim and square toes. 4 6-year-old boy, *c.* 1839. Short cotton jacket, bloused bodice with edge-to-edge fastening, high round neckline with double frill, buttoned-down collar set into bodice from shoulder to shaped waistband, long sleeves with sewn cuffs. Ankle-length trousers in matching fabric. Large brimless beret. Knitted cotton stockings. Heelless cloth pumps. 5 12-year-old boy, *c.* 1839. Knee-length wool coat, single-breasted fitted bodice with braid trim and double-breasted button detail, velvet collar, long tight sleeves. Shirt with high frill-edged collar and matching stock. Ankle-length wool trousers. Silk top hat with curled brim. Heelless cloth boots with leather soles and square toecaps. 6 4-year-old boy, *c.* 1839. Waist-length wool jacket worn open, large pearl button trim, matching trim on sewn cuffs of long sleeves. Cotton shirt with large pointed Peter Pan collar and long sleeves, worn with knotted silk ribbon tie. Ankle-length checked wool trousers. Matching brimless hat with braid trim. Knitted cotton stockings. Heelless cloth shoes with leather soles. 7 4-year-old boy, *c.* 1840. Knee-length velvet dress with wide neckline open to high waist, turned-back silk revers, long leg-of-mutton sleeves, open skirts. Silk blouse with wide frill-edged neckline. Ankle-length cotton drawers. Knitted silk stockings. Heelless leather shoes with ties and square toes.

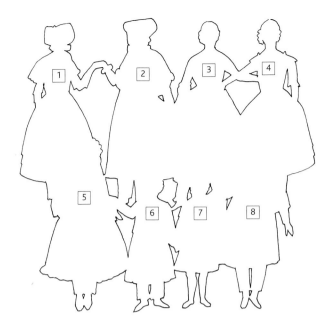

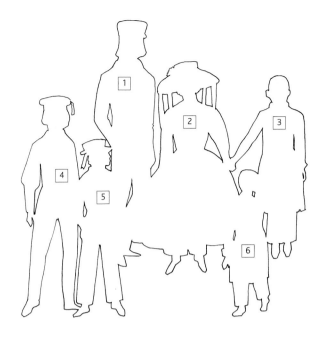

1841–1842

1 8-year-old girl, *c.* 1841. Silk dress with low neckline, fitted bodice with ruched front panel and wide tucked collar to waistline edged with small box-pleats, matching detail at elbow level on long sleeves, full skirt with tucks above hemline. Ankle-length drawers edged with tucks and lace. Bonnet with ruched silk inner brim, crown trimmed with silk flowers and ribbon, bow tie under chin. Cloth gloves. Cloth boots with leather soles and square toecaps. 2 8-year-old girl, *c.* 1842. Single-breasted wool coat with waist-length cape, fur-trimmed hemline, matching collar and cuffs of long sleeves, full skirts. Ankle-length drawers with lace trim. Straw bonnet with silk back frill, ribbon trim, bow tie under chin. Short cloth gloves. Knitted silk stockings. Heelless leather slippers with tied bar straps. 3 8-year-old girl, *c.* 1841. Striped cotton dress, fitted bodice with low V-shaped neckline edged with lace and trimmed with covered buttons, matching ruched hems of three-quarter-length sleeves and edges of open skirt. Ankle-length drawers with frilled hems. Elbow-length crocheted fingerless gloves. Knitted cotton stockings. Heelless kid pumps. 4 8-year-old girl, *c.* 1842. Silk dress, fitted bodice with wide frill-edged neckline, matching hems of elbow-length sleeves, braid-trimmed bodice and sleeves, full skirt with tucks above hemline. Elbow-length crocheted fingerless gloves. Ankle-length cotton drawers with scalloped edge and embroidered detail. 5 6-year-old girl, *c.* 1842. Single-breasted checked wool coat with lace collar, elbow-length cape, long sleeves with button-trimmed sewn cuffs, full skirts. Wool dress with frilled hemline. Ankle-length drawers with lace trim. Bonnet with ruched silk inner brim, ostrich feather trim, ribbon tie under chin. Short crocheted fingerless gloves. Knitted cotton stockings. Heelless leather shoes with tied bar straps. 6 2-year-old boy, *c.* 1841. Patterned silk edge-to-edge waist-length jacket with bound edges, ribbon and ruched silk trim, matching trim above hemline of full skirt, long sleeves gathered into band at wrist. Silk shirt with ruched bodice and plain collar, ribbon tie. Ankle-length drawers trimmed with lace. Heelless cloth boots with leather soles and square toecaps. 7 2-year-old boy, *c.* 1841. Scottish costume: checked wool frock with wide neckline, short sleeves and box-pleated skirt, worn with fringed checked wool stole fastened on one shoulder with a clasp. Large brimless beret with pompon trim. Heelless kid slippers with square toes and ties crisscrossed over knee-length wool stockings. 8 6-year-old boy, *c.* 1842. Loose-fitting velvet frock with large lace-trimmed collar, matching cuffs on leg-of-mutton-style sleeves, centre-front buttoned strap opening, straps repeated on each side of skirt above hemline. Ankle-length wool trousers. Small felt hat with shallow crown and narrow brim. Knitted cotton stockings. Heelless kid pumps with square toes.

1843–1844

1 10-year-old boy, *c.* 1843. Single-breasted waist-length wool jacket, cut to be worn open, button trim on each side, shawl collar and long sleeves with button trim at wrist level. Single-breasted silk waistcoat with shawl collar. Cotton shirt with attached collar, silk scarf knotted at front. Straight-cut wool trousers with stirrups under feet. Wool cap with gathered crown and wide peak. Kid gloves. Leather ankle boots with round toes. 2 9-year-old girl, *c.* 1844. Silk dress, low neckline with gathered gauze in-fill, fitted bodice, gathered checked silk front panel edged with covered buttons, matching epaulettes above leg-of-mutton sleeves and front panel of full skirt. Ankle-length lace-trimmed cotton drawers. Straw hat with shallow crown and wide brim, silk flower and velvet ribbon trim. Cloth boots with leather soles and square toecaps. 3 6-year-old boy, *c.* 1844. Knee-length collarless wool coat, edge-to-edge hook fastening with button trim, matching rows of buttons on each side from shoulder to waist, long sleeves, box-pleated skirts. Ankle-length trousers in matching fabric with tucks above hem. Cotton shirt worn with silk scarf knotted around attached collar, long sleeves with turned-back cuffs. Knitted cotton stockings. Heelless leather pumps with bow ties and square toes. 4 8-year-old boy, *c.* 1843. Striped cotton shirt, tucked bodice with buttoned front strap opening, leg-of-mutton sleeves with buttoned cuffs, plain collar worn with silk bow tie. Straight-cut wool trousers with stirrups under feet, gathered cotton waist-belt with front clasp fastening. Kid gloves. Leather pumps with ties and round toes. 5 6-year-old boy, *c.* 1844. Short wool tweed jacket with cut-away curved front, hook fastening under small stand collar, long sleeves open from elbow level at front, revealing cotton shirt sleeves gathered into narrow cuffs, gathered bodice with frilled neckline worn with knotted silk scarf. Ankle-length striped wool baggy trousers with narrow buttoned waistband. Straw cap, flared crown trimmed with ribbon braid, side bow and ends, wide peak. Heelless cloth boots with leather soles and square toecaps. 6 4-year-old boy, *c.* 1843. Knee-length cotton frock, single-breasted fastening with large pearl buttons under large plain cotton collar, worn with knotted silk scarf, turned-back cuffs under long sleeves matching collar fabric, box-pleated skirt. Ankle-length cotton drawers. Knitted cotton stockings. Heelless leather shoes with bow ties and round toes.

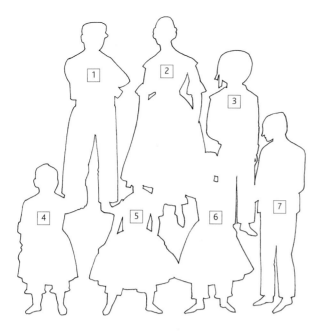

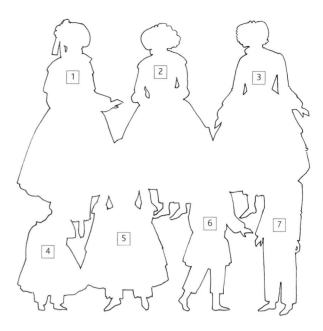

1845–1846

1 5-year-old boy, *c.* 1845. Short single-breasted wool jacket with plain cotton collar, matching cuffs on long sleeves, bow tie. Baggy ankle-length wool trousers with deep waistband buttoned onto jacket. Leather cap with high crown and wide peak. Heelless cloth ankle boots. 2 8-year-old girl, *c.* 1846. Silk dress, fitted bodice with wide neckline, elbow-length sleeves with scalloped frill, matching double epaulettes from shoulder to above ruched panel on front of bodice, full skirt worn over stiffened petticoats. Ankle-length cotton drawers with scalloped frill. Heelless cloth ankle boots with leather soles and square toecaps. 3 6-year-old boy, *c.* 1846. Cotton sailor suit: short bloused top with low neckline, wide contrast-colour collar edged with braid, matching cuffs of long sleeves, under-blouse with large collar and contrast-colour knotted scarf; baggy ankle-length cotton trousers buttoned to blouse. Large straw hat with wide upswept brim and braid trim. Knitted cotton stockings. Heelless Heelless leather pumps with bow trim. 4 2-year-old boy, *c.* 1846. Knee-length velvet frock, fitted bodice with low V-shaped neckline edged with lace collar, wide three-quarter-length cuffed sleeves, mock undersleeves gathered at wrist into frilled hems, narrow self-fabric ruched panels from shoulder to hemline of full skirt. Short cotton drawers with frilled hems. Heelless cloth pumps with leather soles, bow trim and round toes. 5 2-year-old girl, *c.* 1845. Silk dress, fitted bow-trimmed bodice with wide frill-edged neckline, short draped sleeves under epaulettes running from shoulder to centre-front waist, full skirt with panniers and tucked detail above hemline. Short cotton drawers with lace trim. Knitted cotton stockings. Heelless cloth shoes with buttoned bar straps and front detail, round toes. 6 5-year-old girl, *c.* 1846. Cotton dress, fitted bodice with vertical tucked detail and low frill-edged neckline, matching trim on elbow-length sleeves, full skirt with pleated hem detail, worn over petticoats, wide waistband. Ankle-length cotton drawers trimmed with tucks and lace. Heelless cloth ankle boots with leather soles and pointed toecaps. 7 6-year-old boy, *c.* 1845. Hip-length cotton jacket with pearl button fastening, matching trim on long sleeves, shawl collar. Single-breasted cloth waistcoat with shawl collar. Cotton shirt with button fastening, large collar, ribbon bow tie. Ankle-length cotton trousers. Knitted cotton stockings. Heelless leather slippers with square toes.

1847–1849

1 8-year-old girl, *c.* 1849. Mourning clothes: fine wool dress with fitted bodice, three-quarter-length flared sleeves, sham cotton undersleeves gathered into narrow cuffs, full skirt trimmed with velvet ribbon, matching elbow-length cape and sleeves. Plain wool shoulder cape with button fastening and lace collar. Ankle-length cotton drawers with lace trim. Bonnet trimmed with silk flowers and ribbon, bow tie under chin. Short kid gloves. Cloth boots with side-button fastenings and square toecaps. 2 8-year-old girl, *c.* 1848. Wool jacket with fitted bodice, three-quarter-length sleeves with fur cuffs, matching collar, edges and hem of full skirts. Fine wool dress with long sleeves and full skirt with embroidered detail above hemline. Ankle-length cotton drawers with self-fabric pleated hemline. Bonnet with ostrich feathers, silk flowers and ribbon trim, bow tie under chin. Short kid gloves. Heelless cloth boots with side-button fastenings, leather soles, sides and toecaps. 3 8-year-old girl, *c.* 1847. Long silk jacket, fitted bodice with edge-to-edge hooked fastening, three-quarter-length sleeves trimmed with buttons, scalloped cuffs trimmed with lace, matching collar and two rows of trimming on skirts, sham undersleeves with frills. Silk dress, skirt trimmed with bands of self-fabric pleating. Short cotton drawers trimmed with lace. Bonnet trimmed with silk flowers, cords and ribbons, bow tie under chin. Heelless cloth boots with leather soles and toecaps. 4 2-year-old boy, *c.* 1848. Single-breasted checked silk frock with fitted bodice, high neckline with plain silk frill-edged collar, worn with a narrow velvet ribbon bow tie, long sleeves with sewn cuffs, velvet-covered buttons on front fastening, matching button trim on shaped flap pockets on full skirts. Ankle-length cotton drawers. Knitted cotton stockings. Heelless kid shoes with high tongues and round toes. 5 6-year-old girl, *c.* 1849. Silk dress, off-the-shoulder neckline trimmed with lace, matching cuffs on elbow-length ruched sleeves, ruched detail repeated on fitted bodice, three-tier full skirt worn over petticoats. Ankle-length cotton drawers trimmed with lace. Coral necklace. Cloth boots with side-button fastenings, leather soles, sides and square toecaps. 6 4-year-old boy, *c.* 1849. Collarless cotton frock with bloused bodice, centre-front contrast-colour braided buttoned strap fastening, matching trim on three-quarter-length flared sleeves and hemline of full skirt. Cotton shirt with large collar and full sleeves gathered into cuffs. Short cotton drawers with lace trim. Felt hat with shallow crown and wide brim, ribbon rosette and ostrich feather trim. Striped cotton socks. Heelless kid slippers with square toes. 7 5-year-old boy, *c.* 1847. Waist-length wool jacket, worn open, pearl button trim, matching trim on long sleeves. Single-breasted patterned silk waistcoat. Cotton shirt with large collar and long sleeves, silk scarf knotted at front. Ankle-length wool trousers. Knitted cotton stockings. Heelless kid slippers with pointed toes.

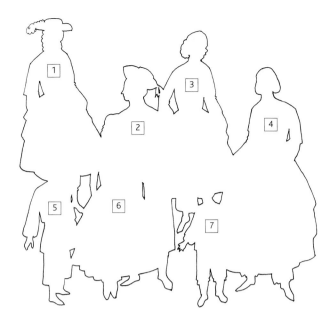

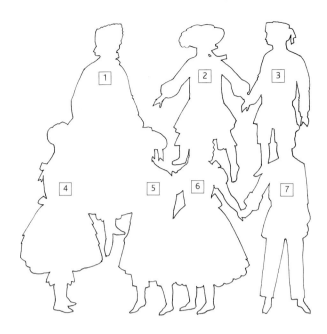

1850–1851

1 6-year-old girl, *c.* 1850. Silk dress, fitted bodice with low square neckline, deep waist-belt and two-tier skirt, all with velvet ribbon trim, matching trim on collarless hip-length open jacket with three-quarter-length flared sleeves, sham undersleeves gathered into cuffs edged with frills. Short cotton drawers gathered into frills. Felt hat with wide-brim crown trimmed with ostrich feathers and ribbons. Heelless cloth boots. 2 9-year-old boy, *c.* 1850. Checked cotton shirt with bodice gathered from yoke under large collar and plain cotton scarf, buttoned strap fastening and long sleeves with buttoned cuffs. Knee-length cotton trousers with fall fronts. Large straw hat with turned-back brim, high crown trimmed with ribbon, tails at back. Striped wool socks. Ankle boots with elastic sides and small heels. 3 6-year-old girl, *c.* 1850. Striped cotton dress, fitted bodice with high round neckline trimmed with lace collar, three-quarter-length flared sleeves with plain cotton sham undersleeves gathered into cuffs, full skirt, cord belt. Cotton drawers gathered into narrow bands at ankle level. Heelless cloth boots with leather soles, sides and pointed toecaps. 4 10-year-old girl, *c.* 1850. Patterned silk dress with fitted bodice, low round neckline in-filled with transparent sham blouse with lace collar and velvet bow, elbow-length sleeves with matching sham undersleeves, three-tier full skirt edges trimmed with velvet ribbon, matching hem of sleeves, neckline and buttons on centre front of bodice. Ankle-length cotton drawers with lace trim. Hair worn in open net cap. Knitted silk stockings. Heelless kid slippers with crossed ribbon ties. 5 4-year-old boy, *c.* 1851. Hip-length cotton blouse with asymmetric button fastening, high neckline with large collar and knotted scarf, long sleeves gathered into cuffs, buckled leather waist-belt. Mid-calf-length cotton trousers. Felt cap with tall crown and leather peak. Knitted socks. Heelless leather slippers with buttoned bar straps and pointed toes. 6 6-year-old girl, *c.* 1851. Patterned silk dress, fitted bodice with button decoration on centre front, braid trim and off-the-shoulder neckline, matching trim on short sleeves, three-tier skirt. Cotton drawers with lace trim. Knitted silk stockings. Heelless kid slippers with buttoned bar straps and square toes. 7 3-year-old boy, *c.* 1850. Single-breasted collarless wool jacket with three-quarter-length sleeves. Cotton blouse, buttoned strap fastening edged with lace frill, matching large collar, worn with bow tie, cuffs on long sleeves and frill on drawers under knee-length wool trousers. Brimless hat trimmed with embroidery, cord and feathers. Knitted cotton stockings. Heelless kid ankle boots with elasticated sides.

1852–1854

1 8-year-old girl, *c.* 1852. Short wool coat, fitted bodice with edge-to-edge hooked fastening, wide collar trimmed with velvet ribbon, matching detail above hems of three-quarter-length flared sleeves, full skirts. Silk dress bands of quilted detail above hemline on full skirt, repeated on hems of three-quarter-length sleeves, sham undersleeves gathered at wrists. Short cotton drawers trimmed with embroidered lace. Bonnet covered with ruched silk, back frill and frilled front edge, lined with contrast-colour ruched silk. Cloth gloves. Knitted silk stockings. Heelless ankle boots with button fastening, leather soles and square toecaps. 2 3-year-old boy, *c.* 1853. Hip-length collarless jacket fastened across front with looped cord and buttons, edges trimmed with fur, matching three-quarter-length sleeves and above hemline of full skirt, sham undersleeves gathered into cuffs. Short cotton drawers with scalloped hemlines. Straw hat with wide brim, ostrich feather and ribbon trimming, bow tie under chin. Knitted cotton socks. Heelless kid ankle boots with elasticated sides. 3 4-year-old boy, *c.* 1854. Cotton suit: hip-length single-breasted collarless jacket with long cuffed sleeves and low-slung buckled belt, matching short trousers, plain cotton collar and knotted scarf. Straw hat with wide turned-back brim and high crown trimmed with ribbon band, matching tails. Knee-length knitted socks. Kid slippers with bar straps. 4 6-year-old girl, *c.* 1853. Striped silk party dress, fitted bodice with off-the-shoulder neckline edged with satin and trimmed with bows, matching bound edges of lace-trimmed tiered skirt, waist-sash and short drawers. Knitted silk stockings. Heelless cloth ankle-length boots with side-laced fastenings, leather soles and toecaps. 5 5-year-old boy, *c.* 1854. Knee-length cotton frock, bodice with lace-edged vertical tucks on each side of button fastening under lace-trimmed collar to waist, long cuffed sleeves, full skirt, wide contrast-colour belt with snake buckle fastening, knotted silk scarf. Short cotton drawers with lace trim. Felt hat with wide brim turned up at front and back, ribbon trim and tails. Knitted socks. Heelless leather boots with front lacings and toecaps. 6 5-year-old girl, *c.* 1852. Silk party dress with low neckline, wide self-binding edged with lace, matching cross-over detail on fitted bodice, bow trim above puff sleeves, wide pleated cummerbund with large bow on one side, long fringed ends, full skirt trimmed with bands of lace. Lace-edged petticoat. Pearl necklace. Heelless cloth boots with button fastenings, leather soles and square toecaps. 7 6-year-old boy, *c.* 1853. Hip-length cotton blouse, bodice with buttoned strap opening edged in braid, matching collar, wide cuffs of three-quarter-length sleeves, buckled belt and hemline, sham sleeves gathered into cuffs. Ankle-length trousers in matching fabric. Cloth cap with band, gathered crown and wide peak. Heelless kid boots with elasticated sides.

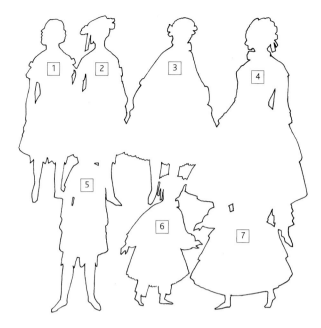

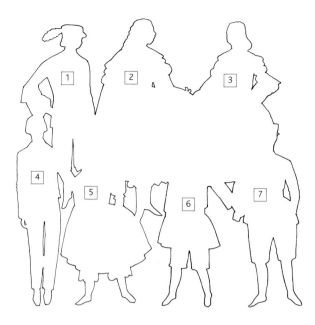

1855–1856

1 5-year-old girl, *c.* 1856. Silk dress with bloused bodice under row of diagonal tucks and lace-edged off-the-shoulder neckline, lace edging repeated on hems of short sleeves below inset satin band, matching satin bow trim on each shoulder and around hipline, three-tier gathered skirt with pinked edges. Short lace drawers. Three-quarter-length knitted socks. Heelless cloth ankle boots with button fastenings, leather soles and square toecaps.

2 5-year-old boy, *c.* 1855. Checked silk frock with short deep cuffed sleeves, open front fastened with jet beaded braid, buttoned across at chest and waist level, matching trim on gathered skirt. Silk blouse with bloused bodice, long cuffed sleeves and large embroidered collar with scalloped edge. Short lace drawers. Velvet hat with narrow brim and gathered crown, ostrich feather and ribbon trim. Heelless knee-length cloth boots with leather soles, sides and fronts.

3 6-year-old girl, *c.* 1856. Collarless edge-to-edge hip-length velvet jacket fastened with hooks, trimmed with bands of brightly coloured pleated silk, matching hems and decoration on elbow-length flared sleeves, sham undersleeves gathered at wrists. Checked silk skirt worn over lace-edged petticoat. Ruched and pleated silk bonnet trimmed with ribbon bows, bow tie under chin. Short kid gloves. Knitted silk stockings. Heelless cloth boots with leather soles and square toecaps.

4 9-year-old girl, *c.* 1855. Silk dress with fitted bodice, low wide neckline filled in with rows of gathered silk, matching hems of flared sleeves with ribbon and lace borders, ribbon and lace trim repeated on wide wrap-over collar and two-tier gathered skirt. Ankle-length frilled cotton drawers. Bonnet with ruched inner brim trimmed with artificial flowers and edged in lace, crown trimmed with loops of silk ribbon, bow tie under chin. Short kid gloves. Heelless cloth boots with leather soles and square toecaps.

5 6-year-old boy, *c.* 1856. Short cotton frock gathered from high yoke, single-breasted button fastening from neck to hem, short sleeves, buckled leather belt. Cotton blouse with scallop-edged collar, worn with bow tie, and long sleeves gathered into cuffs. Knee-length scallop-edged cotton drawers. Long knitted socks. Heelless ankle-length cloth boots with laced fastenings, leather soles and square toecaps.

6 2-year-old boy, *c.* 1855. Striped silk coat with wrist-length fringed cape, lace collar and silk bow tie, sham undersleeves gathered at wrists. Embroidered cotton petticoat and matching drawers. Felt hat with curled brim, crown trimmed with ostrich feathers and ribbon band. Knitted ankle socks. Heelless cloth slippers.

7 6-year-old girl, *c.* 1855. Striped silk dress with fitted bodice, large pleated collar over wide frill-edged neckline, matching frilled cuffs on three-tier puffed sleeves, edge of top tier trimmed with pleated contrast-colour silk, matching waist-sash, bow and edges of three-tier gathered skirt. Knitted stockings. Heelless cloth ankle boots with leather soles and toecaps.

1857–1858

1 6-year-old boy, *c.* 1857. Edge-to-edge hip-length wool jacket fastened with hooks and trimmed with wide ribbon braid, matching hems of three-quarter-length flared sleeves and side seams of lace-trimmed knee-length trousers. Cotton shirt with large collar and long sleeves gathered into cuffs. Stiffened felt hat with curled brim and tall crown trimmed with band, bow and ostrich feather. Short kid gloves. Long striped socks. Heelless leather slippers with high tongues and buckle trim.

2 10-year-old girl, *c.* 1858. Striped silk dress, fitted bodice with centre-front hooked fastenings and button and ribbon trim, high neckline with lace-edged collar and knotted silk scarf, gathered two-tier epaulettes, puffed sleeves above wide flared undersleeves, hems trimmed with self-fabric pleating, bows and lace, three-tier gathered skirt, lace petticoat. Knitted silk stockings. Heelless kid ankle boots.

3 9-year-old girl, *c.* 1857. Checked cotton dress, fitted bodice with vertical tucks, three-quarter-length sleeves, two ruched puffs above circular cuffs trimmed with bands of braid, repeated above hemline of full skirt, high round neckline with plain cotton frilled edge, matching sham undersleeves gathered into cuffs at wrist level. Cotton drawers. Knitted cotton stockings. Ankle-length leather boots with elasticated sides and low heels.

4 5-year-old boy, *c.* 1857. Short collarless jacket with hooked fastening on high neckline, long sleeves with button-trim braid edges, matching trim on pockets and edges of single-breasted waistcoat. Ankle-length trousers in matching fabric. Cotton shirt with long sleeves and large collar, ribbon bow tie. Knitted cotton stockings. Leather slippers with round toes.

5 2-year-old girl, *c.* 1858. Velvet dress, fitted bodice with wide frill-edged neckline, matching hems of short puff sleeves, waist-length collar trimmed with ribbon and jet beads, ribbon trim repeated on edges of hip-length peplum and above hemline of gathered skirt. Scallop-edged embroidered cotton drawers. Knitted silk stockings. Ankle-length leather boots with elasticated sides and low heels.

6 4-year-old boy, *c.* 1857. Hip-length linen jacket with bloused bodice, buttoned strap fastening with velvet ribbon trimming, matching trim above wrists on long sleeves, edges of collar, detail on full skirt and knee-length trousers, self-fabric belt with snake buckle, scallop-edged cotton collar, matching pleated hem detail on sleeves and trousers. Knitted stockings. Leather shoes with buttoned bar straps and round toes.

7 5-year-old boy, *c.* 1858. Hip-length wool tweed collarless jacket with single-breasted leather button fastening, long sleeves with leather trim, matching buckled belt, knee-length breeches in self-fabric, lace frills at neckline and sleeve hems, velvet ribbon bow tie. Leather cap with high crown and wide peak. Knee-length cloth gaiters with stirrups under heelless leather slippers with round toes.

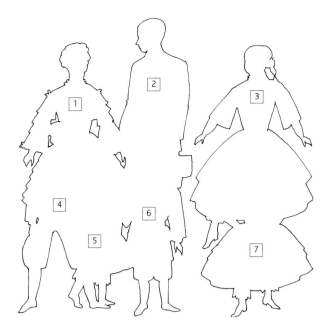

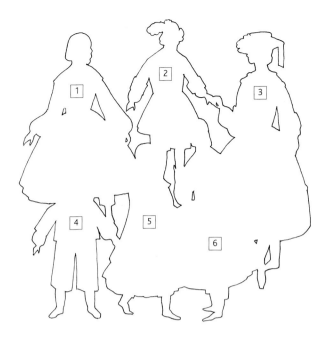

1859–1861

1 8-year-old girl, c. 1860. Checked silk dress, fitted bodice with row of buttons, yoke seams from edge of shoulder to centre-front waist, edged with self-fabric pleats, three-quarter-length tiered sleeves, full skirt finished with five tiers of frills, plain fabric flared undersleeves edged with self-fabric pleats, matching pleated frill around high neckline. 2 10-year-old boy, c. 1861. Short single-breasted wool jacket with wide collar and revers, long sleeves, stitched cuffs and top-stitched edges and detail. Single-breasted collarless wool waistcoat with top-stitched edges. Cotton shirt with stiff collar, worn with silk bow tie. Wool trousers with fall fronts. Felt top hat with curled brim. 3 8-year-old girl, c. 1860. Plain silk dress with fitted bodice, low square neckline, full skirt edged with jet beads, matching wide hems of three-quarter-length checked silk sleeves, underskirt in matching fabric. Silk gauze blouse with high neckline edged with self-fabric pleats, long tight sleeves with button fastenings. Scallop-edged cotton drawers. Silk ribbon bow in hair. Knitted cotton stockings. Ankle-length cloth boots with leather soles, toecaps and low heels. 4 7-year-old boy, c. 1860. Three-piece linen suit: short jacket with hook fastening under large plain cotton shirt collar, long sleeves with contrast-colour braid and button trimming, matching jacket fronts and edges of single-breasted waistcoat; knee-length breeches. Straw hat with wide brim, crown trimmed with ribbon and bow. Striped knitted cotton stockings. Leather slippers with buckle trim, round toes and low heels. 5 2-year-old boy, c. 1860. Striped wool frock, centre-front fastening with large contrast-colour buttons, matching binding on short sleeves and inset band above hemline of skirt, plain cotton scallop-edged collar and sleeve trim. Cotton drawers with scalloped hem. Short socks. Heelless cloth boots with elasticated sides. 6 2-year-old boy, c. 1859. Long linen jacket, strap and button fastening edged with braid, matching decoration on bloused bodice, skirt, long flared sleeves, wide waist-belt and side seams of knee-length breeches. Plain cotton shirt with long sleeves gathered at wrist level, large collar worn with silk bow tie. Striped knitted cotton stockings. Heelless ankle-length cloth boots with button fastenings, square toecaps and leather soles. 7 6-year-old girl, c. 1859. Striped silk dress, fitted bodice with inset tuck on each side from shoulder to centre-front waist, button trim under lace collar, elbow-length sleeves with tucks, matching tucks above hemline of full skirt. Cotton drawers with lace trim. Striped knitted cotton stockings. Ankle-length kid boots with button fastenings, pointed toecaps and low heels.

1862–1863

1 8-year-old girl, c. 1862. Single-breasted fine wool coat, fitted bodice with velvet-covered buttons through to hemline of full skirts, matching wide lapels, edges of epaulettes and hems of shaped flared sleeves. Cotton blouse with tucked bodice, buttoned strap fastening, long sleeves gathered into cuffs, ribbon bow tie at neck. Lace-trimmed cotton drawers. Hair secured in open net at back. Striped knitted cotton stockings. Ankle-length kid boots with button fastenings and square toecaps. 2 3-year-old boy, c. 1863. Single-breasted collarless corded velvet jacket, three-quarter-length sleeves with wide cuffs decorated with fancy braid, matching hip-level pockets, hemline of full skirts and hems of knee-length trousers. Cotton shirt with tiny collar and long sleeves gathered into cuffs, ribbon bow tie at neck. Felt hat with curled brim and domed crown, ostrich feather and braid trimmings. Striped knitted cotton stockings. Ankle-length boots. 3 12-year-old girl, c. 1863. Silk dress with row of covered buttons in contrast fabric on centre front of fitted bodice, matching fabric of ruched trimming on either side of front, on flared hems of sleeves and in garlands above hemline of full skirt, tiny collar, matching sham undersleeves gathered into cuffs. Straw hat with wide brim and shallow crown, ostrich feather and silk ribbon trimmings. Striped knitted cotton stockings. Cloth ankle boots with button fastenings, leather soles, square toecaps and low heels. 4 3-year-old boy, c. 1862. Edge-to-edge collarless silk jacket, front edges and hems trimmed with lace, repeated on three-quarter-length sleeves and on side seams of mid-calf-length matching trousers. Silk shirt with small collar, tucked bodice with buttoned strap fastening, long sleeves gathered into cuffs. Short socks. Heelless cloth boots with leather soles, sides and fronts. 5 5-year-old girl, c. 1862. Three-quarter-length fur coat with flared sleeves and large hood with tassel trim. Fur hand muff in contrast colour. Full skirt. Plain drawers. Cloth bonnet gathered into frill at back, tucked brim trimmed with lace, ribbon tie under chin. Knitted cotton stockings. Ankle-length kid boots with small heels and toecaps in contrast colour. 6 7-year-old girl, c. 1863. Silk dress, fitted bodice with high neckline, sham undersleeves, three-quarter-length flared sleeves and full skirt trimmed with fancy braid and jet beads. Plain drawers. Ankle-length cloth boots with leather soles, toecaps and small heels.

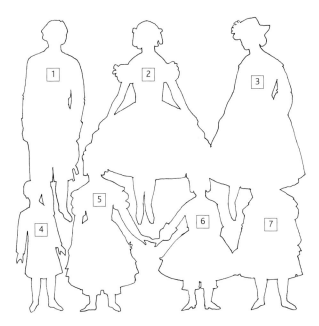

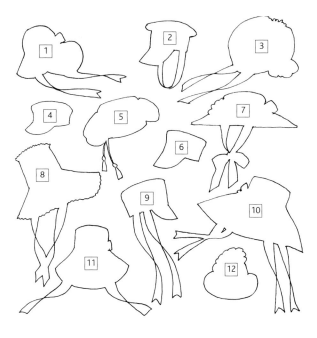

1864 –1866

1 6-year-old boy, *c.* 1865. Long linen jacket, long sleeves with shaped cuffs, strap and brass button fastening from under small collar, matching single button fastening on wide belt and trim on side seams of knee-length trousers, top-stitched edges and detail. Cotton shirt with small collar and long sleeves. Dyed straw hat with wide brim and shallow crown, ribbon band and bow trim. Knitted cotton stockings. Long leather boots with tassel trim, round toes and low heels. 2 6-year-old girl, *c.* 1866. Silk party dress, fitted bodice with short puff sleeves and low off-the-shoulder neckline trimmed with ruched self-fabric, ribbon bows and silk flowers, matching trimmings on hemline of swagged overskirt held by long cords with tasselled ends, cord detail repeated on edges of wide ruched self-fabric cummerbund, underskirt of contrast-colour striped silk. Bow hair decorations. Pearl necklace with crucifix. Knitted silk stockings. Silk slippers with silk rosette trim. 3 7-year-old girl, *c.* 1865. Silk bolero-style jacket edged with contrast-colour satin and beaded braid, matching epaulettes, hems of flared sleeves and bands of decoration above hemline of full skirt, wide belt and shaped buckle edged with matching satin. Silk blouse with small collar and long sleeves gathered into cuffs. Straw hat with wide brim and high crown, feather and satin ribbon trim. Short kid gloves. Knitted silk stockings. Ankle-length cloth boots with scalloped side-button fastening, leather soles and square toecaps. 4 2-year-old boy, *c.* 1866. Long single-breasted wool jacket with front edges and hem, small collar, trim and sewn cuffs on long sleeves, patch pockets and detail on front of knee-length skirt bound and trimmed to match in contrast-colour wool. Cotton shirt collar with cord tie fastening. Striped knitted cotton stockings. Heelless ankle-length cloth boots with round toes and leather soles. 5 3-year-old girl, *c.* 1865. Silk dress with fitted bodice, wide neckline edged with contrast-colour frill, shoulder-wide collar with scalloped edge above two-tier puff sleeves trimmed with rows of velvet ribbon braid, matching wide belt, hem, frills and rosettes on overskirt and hem of underskirt. Cotton petticoat with pleated hem, matching drawers. Brimless felt hat with ribbon and feather trim. Knitted silk stockings. Heelless kid ankle-length boots with open laced fronts. 6 2-year-old girl, *c.* 1864. Silk dress, fitted bodice with sham jacket edged with ribbon, braid and pleated frill, matching high neckline, wide cuffs on three-quarter-length sleeves worn over sham undersleeves, pointed belt under pin-tucked upper bodice and rosettes, trim and hemline of full skirt. Cotton drawers with pleated hems. Felt hat with curled brim and shallow crown, braid and feather trim. Knitted cotton stockings. Short kid boots with square toecaps and low patent-leather heels. 7 2-year-old boy, *c.* 1864. Hip-length checked wool jacket with buttoned strap fastening edged with contrast-colour braid, matching off-the-shoulder neckline, circular-cut epaulettes and strap fastening on front of knee-length box-pleated skirt. Cotton shirt with frill-edged V-shaped neckline, puff sleeves above long sleeves gathered at wrist level into pointed frills. Brimless wool hat trimmed with braid. Knitted cotton stockings. Heelless kid ankle boots.

Hats 1800 –1866

1 4-year-old girl, *c.* 1805. Natural straw bonnet with wide brim front and back shaped down on either side, tall rounded crown, satin ribbon band, matching central bow trimming and long attached ribbons to fasten under chin. 2 8-year-old boy, *c.* 1830. Linen and leather cap, tall stiffened linen crown with gathered top, leather band, chinstrap attached with button on either side, matching wide leather peak. 3 8-year-old girl, *c.* 1851. Silk-covered bonnet, wide brim with ruched edging piped and bound with contrast-colour silk, matching back of round button-trimmed crown above wide back frill, upper brim decorated with silk flowers, leaves and bows, long ribbons attached on either side to fasten under chin. 4 4-year-old boy, *c.* 1800. Fine wool cap, wide band with gathered top and wide rounded peak. 5 7-year-old boy, *c.* 1824. Brimless striped velvet cap, wide band with large gathered top, cord and tassel trimming from middle of crown. 6 8-year-old boy, *c.* 1855. Leather cap with tall flat-topped crown, narrow band buttoned on either side, wide rounded peak, top-stitched edges, seams and detail. 7 5-year-old boy, *c.* 1845. Felt hat with wide brim and tall flat-topped crown, velvet ribbon band and bow and tail trimming at back, matching long ribbon attached on either side to tie under chin, ostrich feather trim across front of crown and brim. 8 6-year-old girl, *c.* 1803. Silk-covered bonnet, tall stiffened crown with flat top, edged with contrast-colour pleated frill, matching double frill on edge of wide brim, ribbon band and long ribbons attached on either side to fasten under chin. 9 8-year-old boy, *c.* 1844. Unlined natural straw cap, tall flared crown with flat top, matching rounded peak, satin ribbon band with long ribbon attached on either side to fasten under chin. 10 10-year-old girl, *c.* 1858. Natural straw hat with wide brim, shallow crown banded with and crossed with silk ribbon extended into long ends to tie under chin or be left loose, matching looped ribbons among silk flower decoration on front of hat and matching binding on wired brim. 11 4-year-old boy, *c.* 1810. Natural straw hat with wide turned-down brim and tall flat-topped crown banded with wide satin ribbon and side bow trim, matching long ribbons from either side of inside brim to tie under chin. 12 6-year-old boy, *c.* 1866. Felt hat with tall rounded crown banded with contrast-colour satin ribbon and trimmed with ostrich feather on one side above large satin ribbon bow and rosette, matching binding on edge of narrow curled brim.

Hats 1867–1882

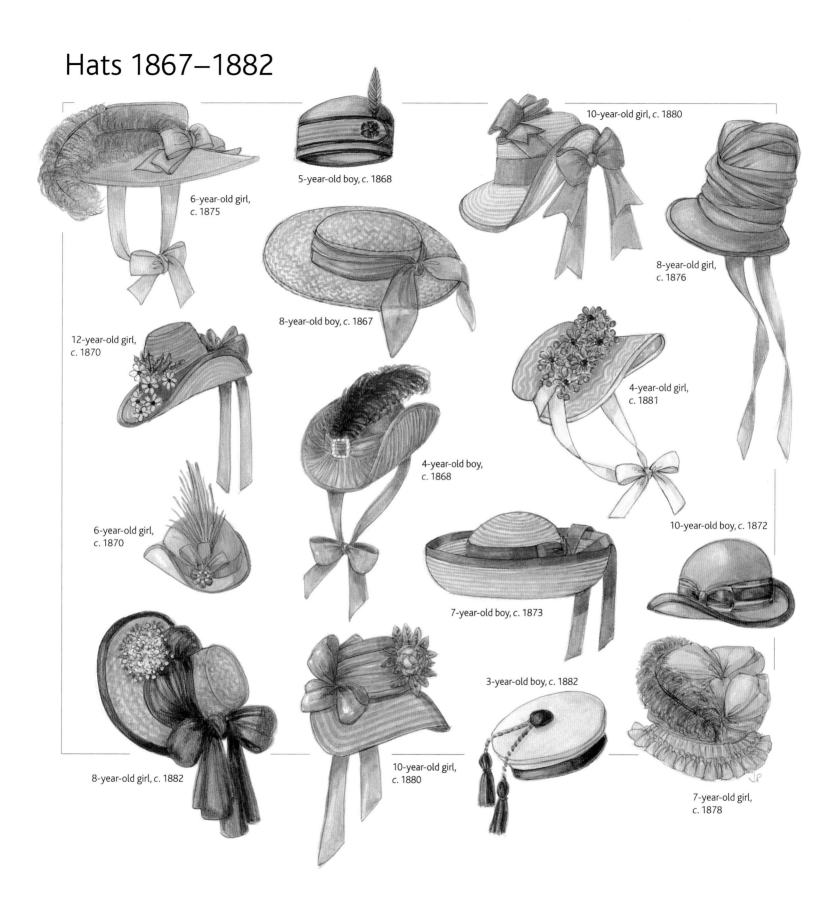

6-year-old girl,
c. 1875

5-year-old boy, c. 1868

10-year-old girl, c. 1880

8-year-old girl,
c. 1876

12-year-old girl,
c. 1870

8-year-old boy, c. 1867

4-year-old girl,
c. 1881

4-year-old boy,
c. 1868

6-year-old girl,
c. 1870

10-year-old boy, c. 1872

7-year-old boy, c. 1873

8-year-old girl, c. 1882

10-year-old girl,
c. 1880

3-year-old boy, c. 1882

7-year-old girl,
c. 1878

1867–1869

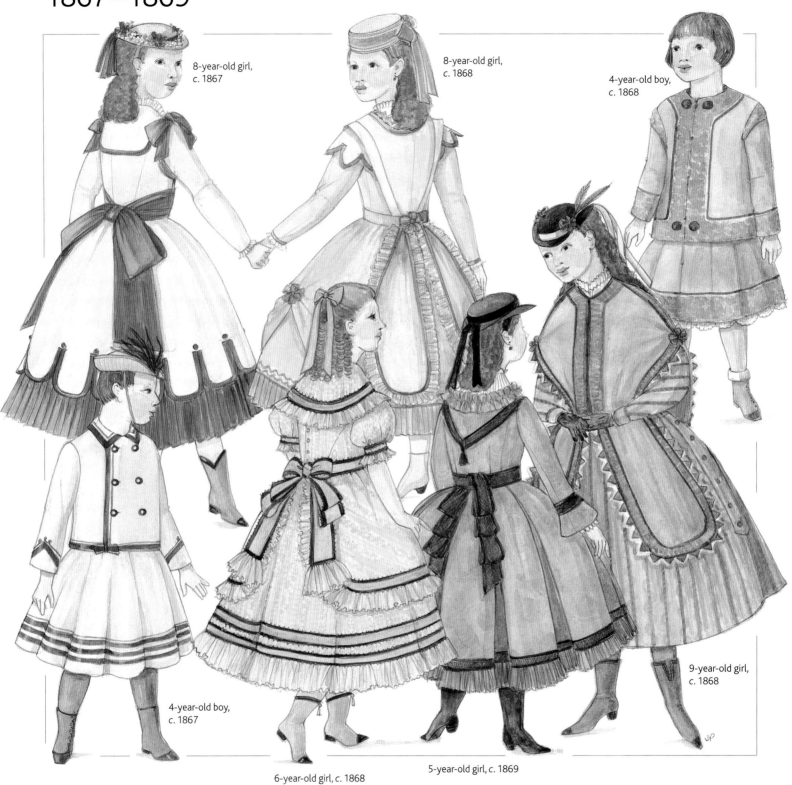

8-year-old girl,
c. 1867

8-year-old girl,
c. 1868

4-year-old boy,
c. 1868

4-year-old boy,
c. 1867

6-year-old girl, c. 1868

5-year-old girl, c. 1869

9-year-old girl,
c. 1868

1870–1872

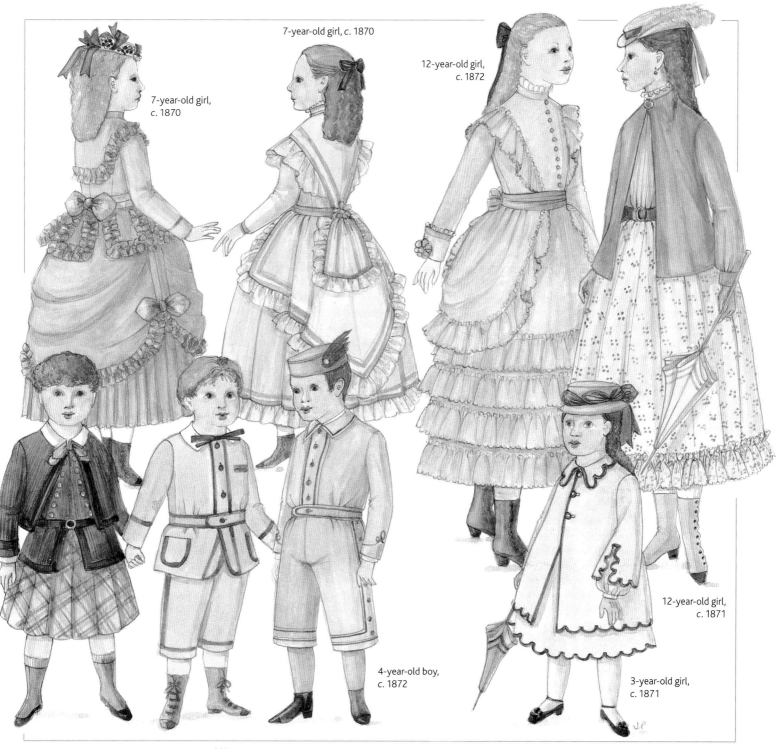

7-year-old girl, c. 1870

7-year-old girl, c. 1870

12-year-old girl, c. 1872

4-year-old boy, c. 1872

4-year-old boy, c. 1871

4-year-old boy, c. 1871

12-year-old girl, c. 1871

3-year-old girl, c. 1871

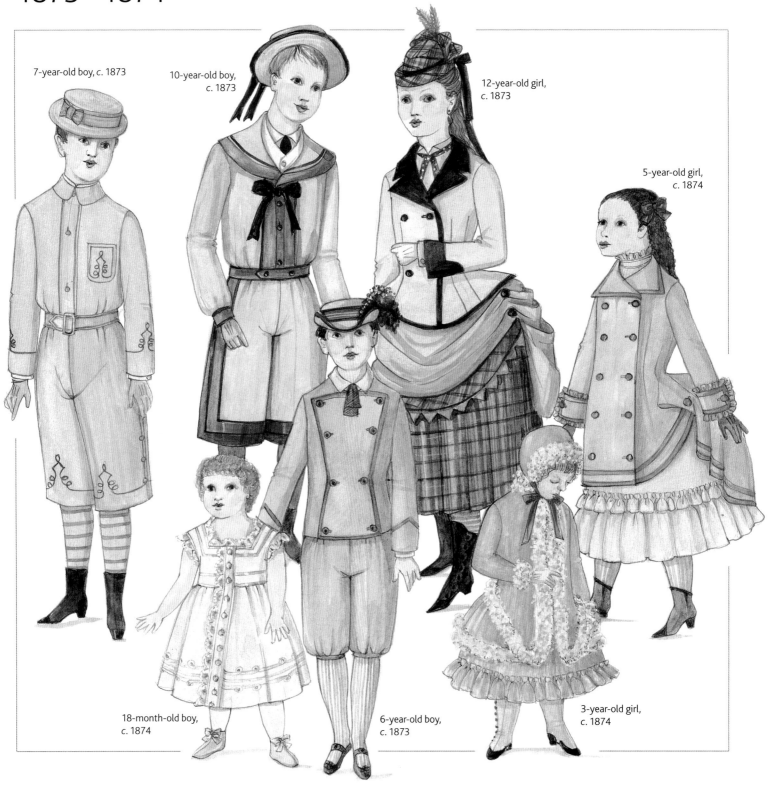

7-year-old boy, *c.* 1873

10-year-old boy, *c.* 1873

12-year-old girl, *c.* 1873

5-year-old girl, *c.* 1874

18-month-old boy, *c.* 1874

6-year-old boy, *c.* 1873

3-year-old girl, *c.* 1874

1875–1877

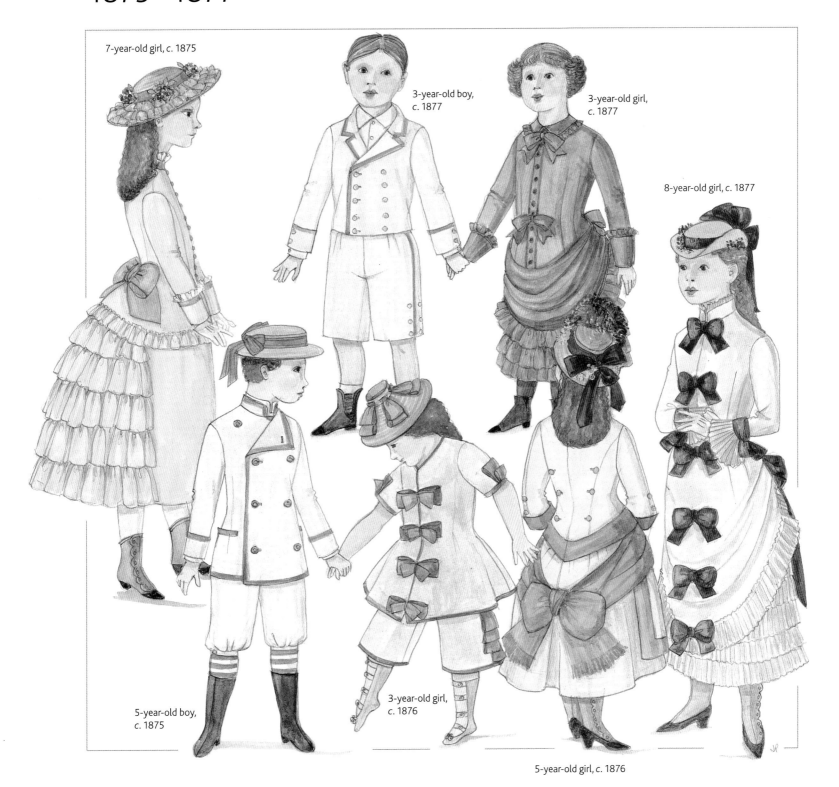

7-year-old girl, *c.* 1875

3-year-old boy, *c.* 1877

3-year-old girl, *c.* 1877

8-year-old girl, *c.* 1877

5-year-old boy, *c.* 1875

3-year-old girl, *c.* 1876

5-year-old girl, *c.* 1876

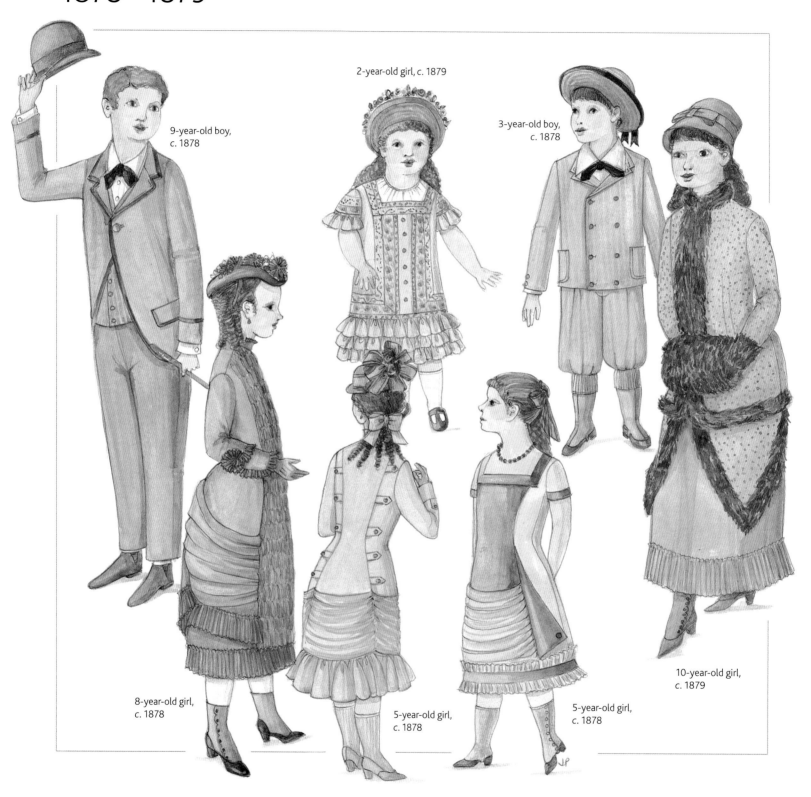

9-year-old boy,
c. 1878

2-year-old girl, c. 1879

3-year-old boy,
c. 1878

8-year-old girl,
c. 1878

5-year-old girl,
c. 1878

5-year-old girl,
c. 1878

10-year-old girl,
c. 1879

1880–1881

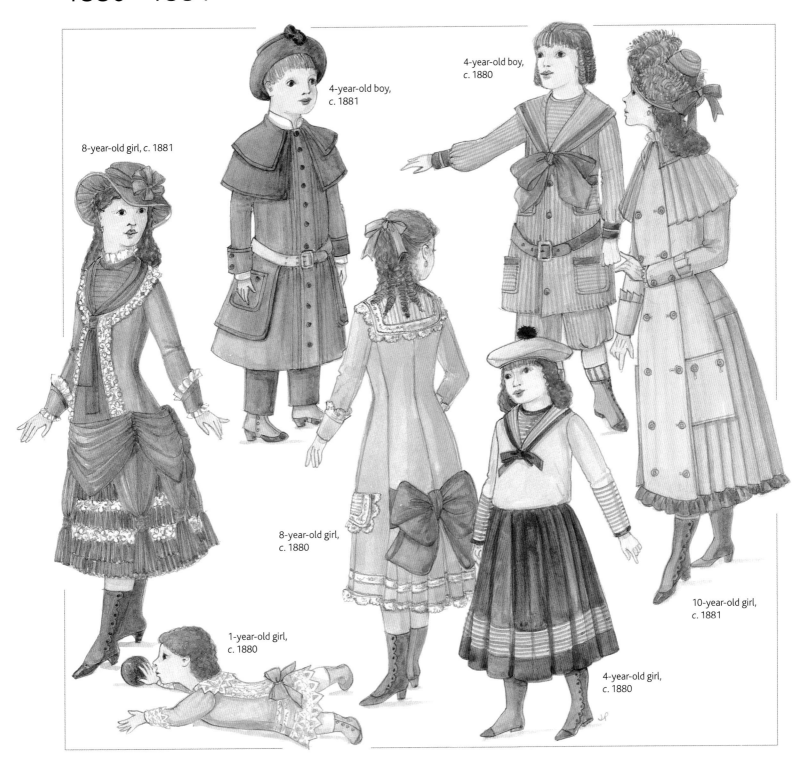

8-year-old girl, c. 1881

4-year-old boy, c. 1881

4-year-old boy, c. 1880

8-year-old girl, c. 1880

1-year-old girl, c. 1880

4-year-old girl, c. 1880

10-year-old girl, c. 1881

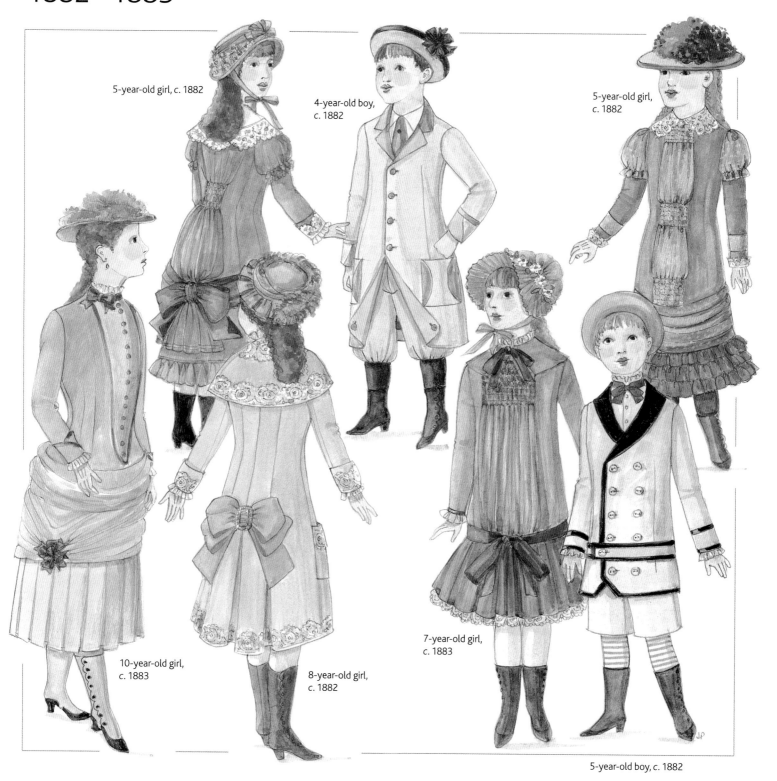

5-year-old girl, c. 1882

4-year-old boy, c. 1882

5-year-old girl, c. 1882

10-year-old girl, c. 1883

8-year-old girl, c. 1882

7-year-old girl, c. 1883

5-year-old boy, c. 1882

1884—1885

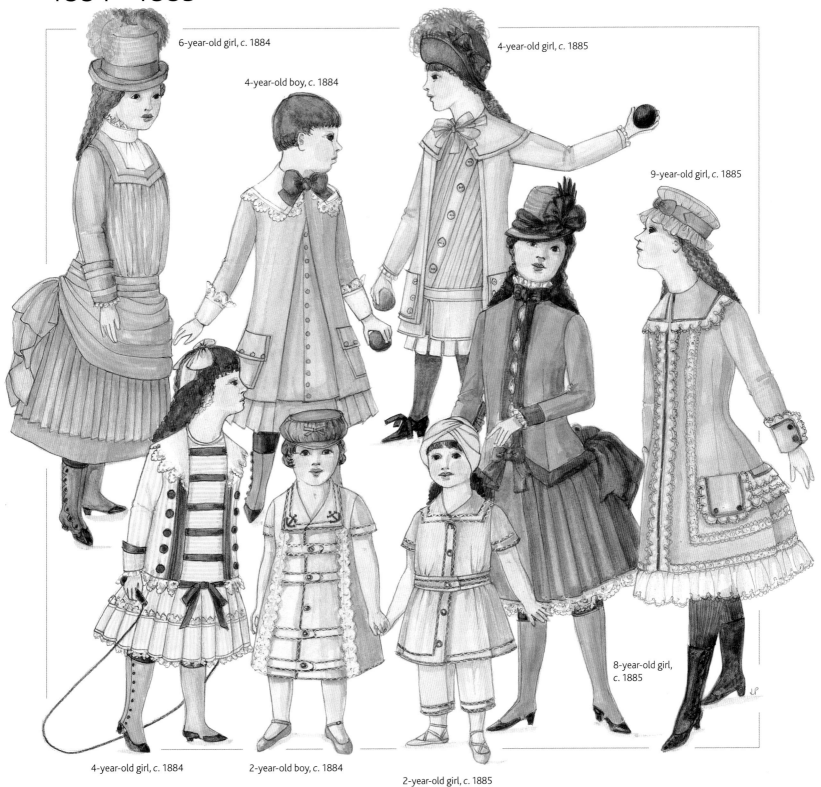

6-year-old girl, c. 1884

4-year-old boy, c. 1884

4-year-old girl, c. 1885

9-year-old girl, c. 1885

8-year-old girl, c. 1885

4-year-old girl, c. 1884

2-year-old boy, c. 1884

2-year-old girl, c. 1885

1886 –1887

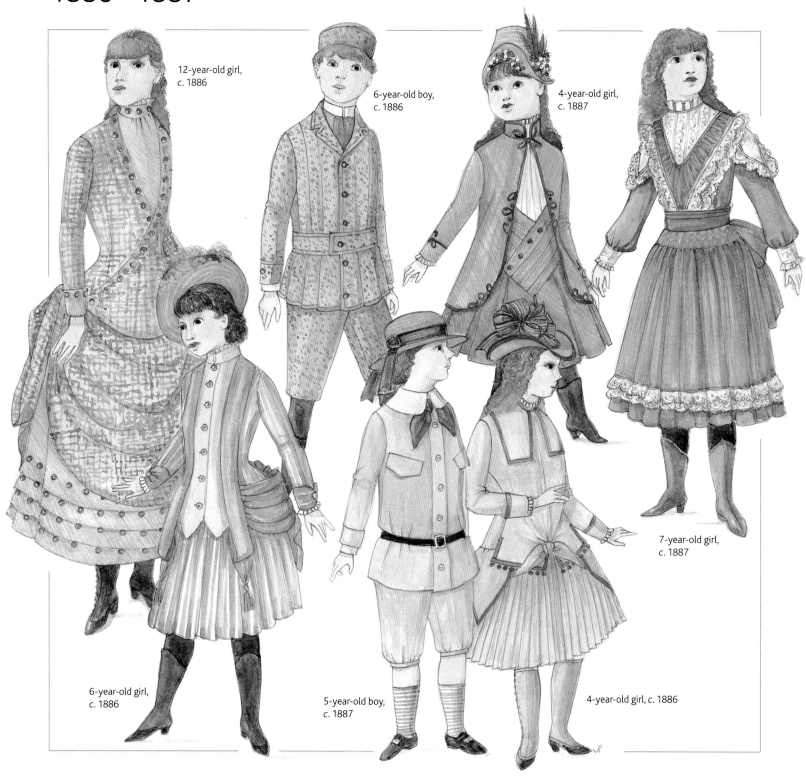

12-year-old girl,
c. 1886

6-year-old boy,
c. 1886

4-year-old girl,
c. 1887

7-year-old girl,
c. 1887

6-year-old girl,
c. 1886

5-year-old boy,
c. 1887

4-year-old girl, *c.* 1886

1888 –1889

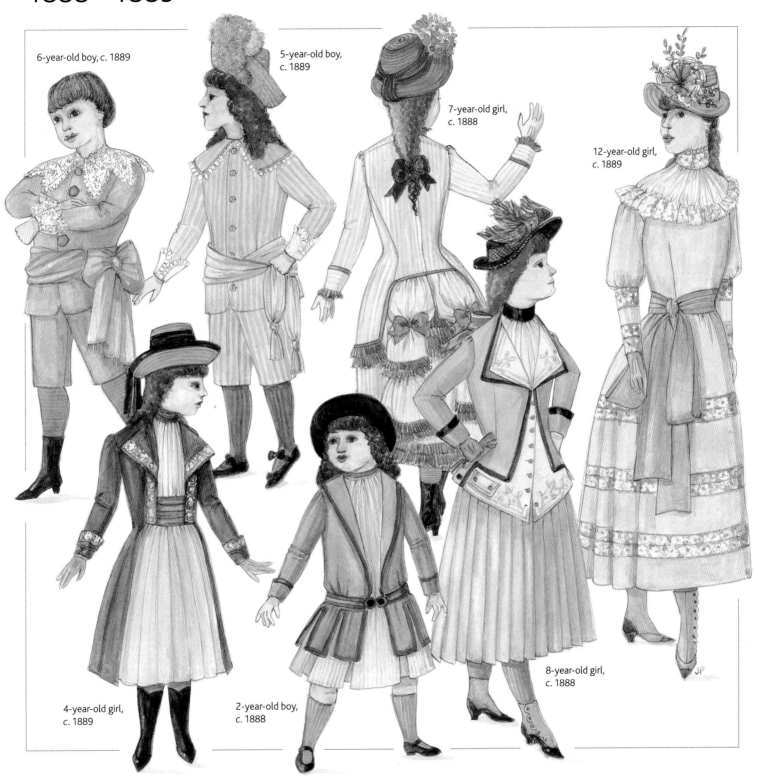

6-year-old boy, c. 1889

5-year-old boy, c. 1889

7-year-old girl, c. 1888

12-year-old girl, c. 1889

4-year-old girl, c. 1889

2-year-old boy, c. 1888

8-year-old girl, c. 1888

1890–1891

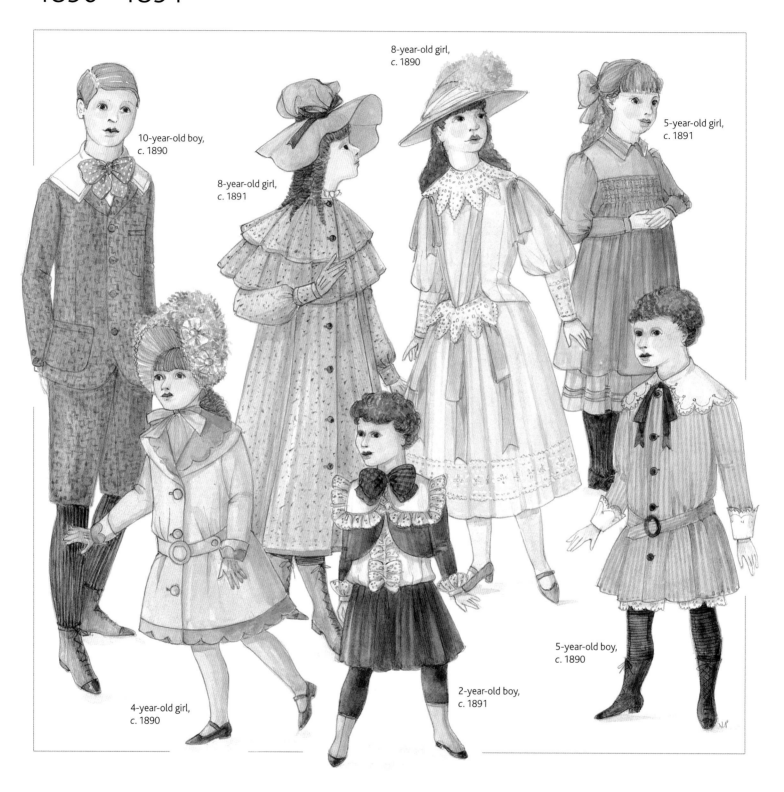

10-year-old boy,
c. 1890

8-year-old girl,
c. 1891

8-year-old girl,
c. 1890

5-year-old girl,
c. 1891

4-year-old girl,
c. 1890

2-year-old boy,
c. 1891

5-year-old boy,
c. 1890

1892–1894

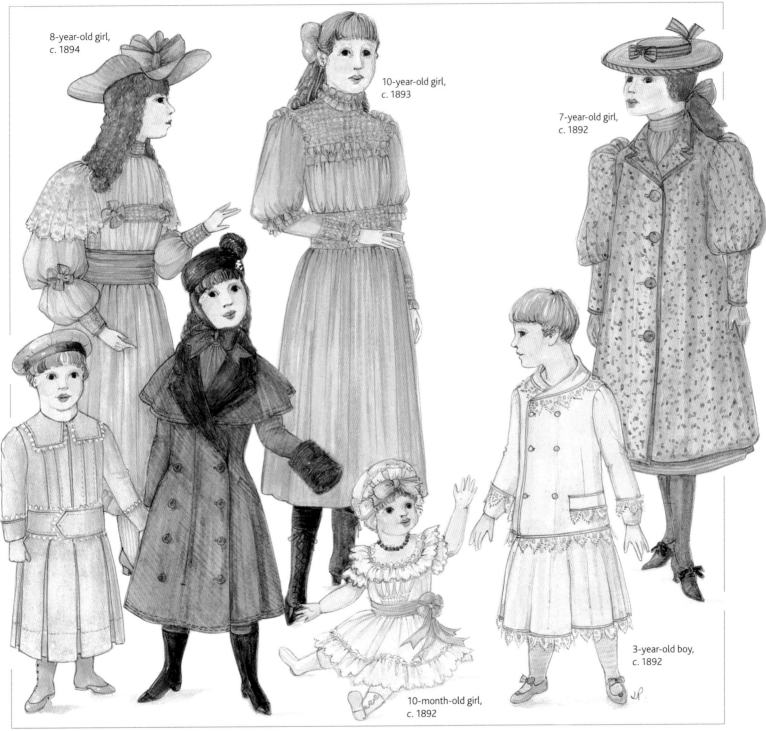

8-year-old girl,
c. 1894

10-year-old girl,
c. 1893

7-year-old girl,
c. 1892

10-month-old girl,
c. 1892

3-year-old boy,
c. 1892

2-year-old boy, c. 1893

5-year-old girl, c. 1894

1895–1896

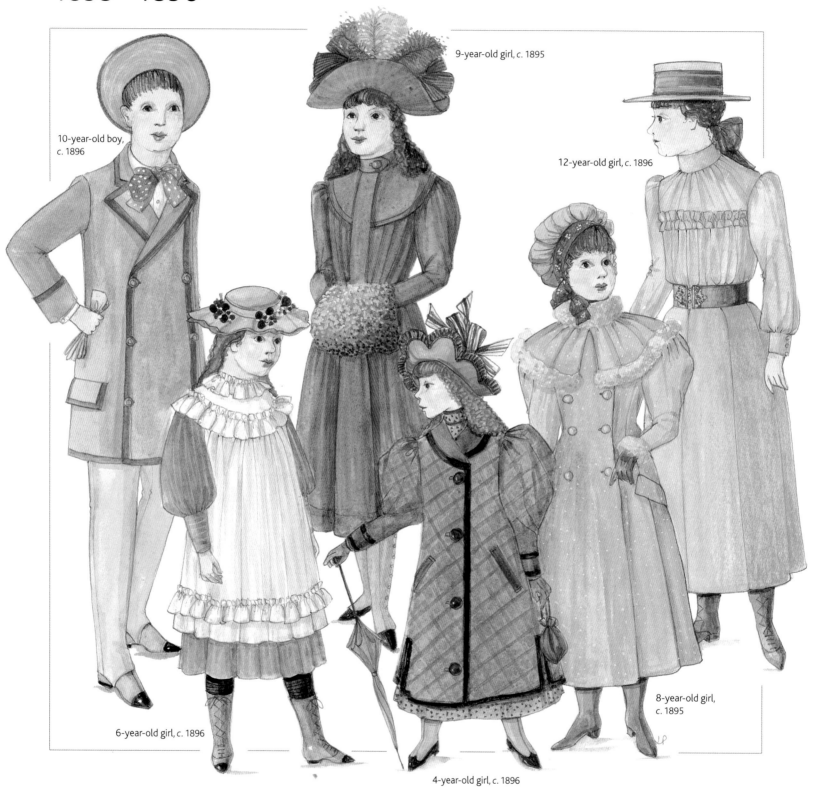

10-year-old boy, *c.* 1896

9-year-old girl, *c.* 1895

12-year-old girl, *c.* 1896

6-year-old girl, *c.* 1896

4-year-old girl, *c.* 1896

8-year-old girl, *c.* 1895

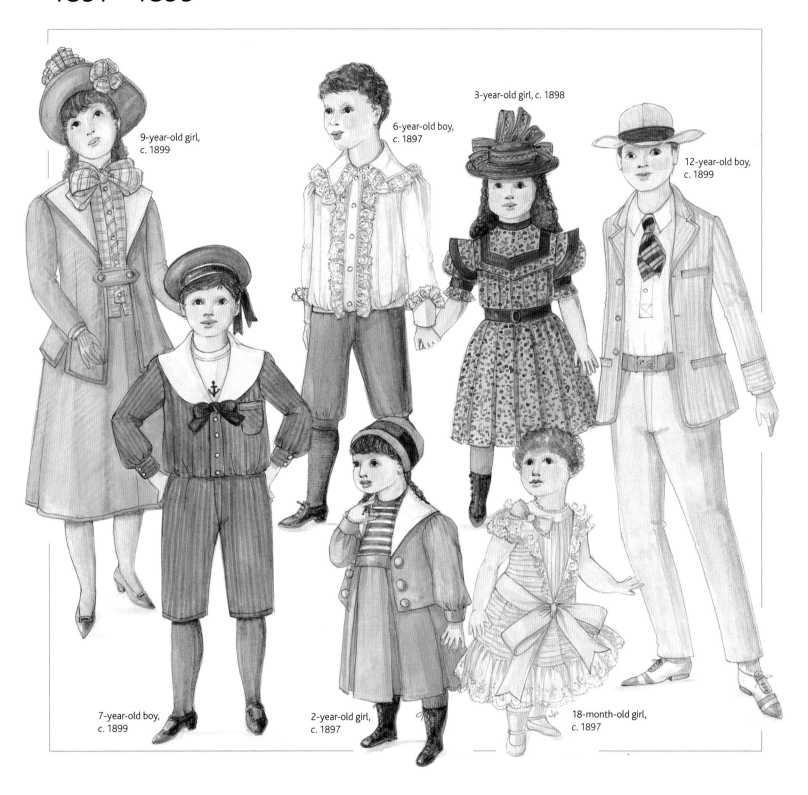

9-year-old girl,
c. 1899

6-year-old boy,
c. 1897

3-year-old girl, c. 1898

12-year-old boy,
c. 1899

7-year-old boy,
c. 1899

2-year-old girl,
c. 1897

18-month-old girl,
c. 1897

Hats 1883–1899

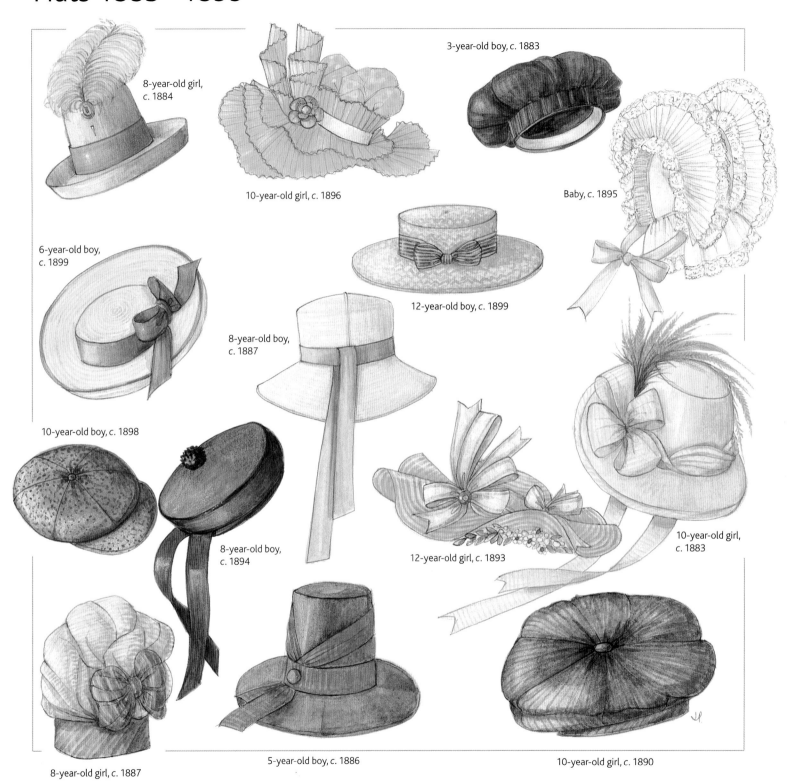

8-year-old girl, *c.* 1884

10-year-old girl, *c.* 1896

3-year-old boy, *c.* 1883

Baby, *c.* 1895

6-year-old boy, *c.* 1899

12-year-old boy, *c.* 1899

8-year-old boy, *c.* 1887

10-year-old boy, *c.* 1898

8-year-old boy, *c.* 1894

12-year-old girl, *c.* 1893

10-year-old girl, *c.* 1883

8-year-old girl, *c.* 1887

5-year-old boy, *c.* 1886

10-year-old girl, *c.* 1890

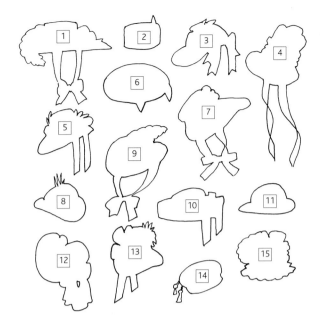

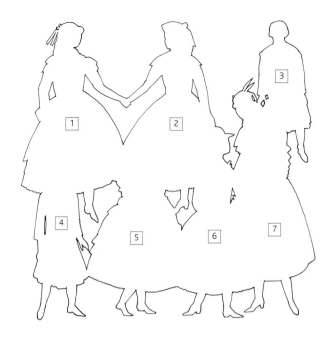

Hats 1867–1882

1 6-year-old girl, *c.* 1875. Silk-covered hat, wide brim with contrast-colour binding, matching colour of ostrich feather trimming on tall crown, large velvet looped ribbon bow set on front, matching ribbons from inside crown with bow tie under chin. 2 5-year-old boy, *c.* 1868. Brimless cloth hat, tall domed crown with contrast-colour bound edge, matching binding on edges of straw band and rosette detail under cut feather trim. 3 10-year-old girl, *c.* 1880. Natural straw hat with wide brim turned up at back of tall crown and held in place by large velvet ribbon bow with long trailing ends, matching band, looped trim on top of crown and bound edges. 4 8-year-old girl, *c.* 1876. Silk bonnet, narrow brim with self-bound edge, tall crown swathed in self-fabric, long silk ribbon ties from inside crown. 5 12-year-old girl, *c.* 1870. Tiny natural straw hat worn on front of head, narrow brim turned up on either side and bound with silk, matching band on tall crown, loops and trailing ends at back, decorative silk flowers and leaves at front. 6 8-year-old boy, *c.* 1867. Natural straw hat, wide flat brim and shallow crown banded with silk scarf, knotted at back. 7 4-year-old girl, *c.* 1881. Fancy-weave natural straw bonnet with wide front brim narrowing at back, edge bound with silk, matching band on shallow crown and long ribbons with bow tie under chin, decorative silk flowers and berries at front. 8 6-year-old girl, *c.* 1870. Tiny stiffened felt hat with narrow brim curled on either side, contrast-colour silk binding, matching loops and rosette trim to one side of narrow band on domed crown, colour repeated in dyed feather spray above. 9 4-year-old boy, *c.* 1868. Ruched silk-covered hat with wide brim curled on either side, contrast-colour binding, matching ruched band on domed crown and ribbons from inside to bow tie under chin, large ostrich feather from above fancy buckle on front. 10 7-year-old boy, *c.* 1873. Natural straw hat with wide brim turned up on front, back and sides, wide silk-bound edge, matching ribbon band on domed crown and bow trim with trailing ends at back. 11 10-year-old boy, *c.* 1872. Stiffened felt hat, narrow curled brim with petersham-bound edge, tall domed crown with striped silk ribbon band and bow to one side. 12 8-year-old girl, *c.* 1882. Fancy-weave natural straw bonnet with wide brim narrowing to back, edge bound with silk, matching scarf tied into large bow at back of tall flat-topped crown, posy of silk flowers set on one side. 13 10-year-old girl, *c.* 1880. Natural straw hat with wide brim turned down at front and up at back, tall flat-topped crown with draped silk band, matching loops, trailing ends and flower set to one side above brim. 14 3-year-old boy, *c.* 1882. Brimless cloth hat with two-piece flat-topped crown set onto narrow contrast-colour petersham band, matching colour of outsized central button and corded tassel trim. 15 7-year-old girl, *c.* 1878. Silk hat with narrow ruched and frill-edged brim, large ruched crown trimmed with ostrich feather in matching colour.

1867–1869

1 8-year-old girl, *c.* 1867. Silk dress with fitted bodice, long tight sleeves with pleated hems, repeated around high neckline of in-fill blouse, low scooped neckline and sleeve heads of dress bound with contrast-colour, matching scalloped hemline with button trim on overskirt, pleated underskirt, wide waist-sash with large bow at back and bow trim on each shoulder. Small straw hat with narrow brim, shallow crown trimmed with flowers, looped ribbons and trailing ribbons at back. Long canvas boots with leather-trimmed shaped tops, pointed toecaps and low heels. 2 8-year-old girl, *c.* 1868. Silk dress with fitted bodice, low neckline bound with contrast-colour velvet, matching edges of scalloped epaulettes, hems of long sleeves above pleated frills, rosette trim on velvet waist-belt and sides of looped-up overskirt and on inner edges of false bow ends at back, contrast-colour silk underskirt with pleated hemline, detail repeated on edges of false bow ends. Brimless straw hat trimmed with wide velvet ribbon, large bow at back and long trailing ends. Knitted silk stockings. Ankle-length kid boots with low heels. 3 4-year-old boy, *c.* 1868. Hip-length collarless wool coat, edge-to-edge front hook fastening trimmed with two buttons on each side of neck and hem, edged with fur and narrow braid, matching epaulettes, cuffs of long sleeves and hem of knee-length full skirt in matching fabric. Cotton petticoat with embroidered scalloped hemline. Short socks rolled over cloth ankle-length boots with side-button fastenings, leather soles, square toecaps and low heels. 4 4-year-old boy, *c.* 1867. Double-breasted linen jacket, high neckline with small collar and long sleeves, full knee-length skirt in matching fabric, edges, bindings, braids and trim in contrast colour. Small fabric-covered hat with turned-up brim and low crown trimmed with feathers. Long knitted cotton stockings. Cloth boots with button fastenings, leather soles, heels and square toecaps. 5 6-year-old girl, *c.* 1868. Striped silk dress, fitted bodice with button fastening at back, shoulder-wide frill-edged collar trimmed with velvet braid, matching cuffs of short puff sleeves, edges of decorative apron, hemline of full skirt and ends of ribbon bow decoration on back of waist-belt. Silk ribbon bow worn in hair at back. Cloth boots with leather soles, heels, pointed toecaps and tassel-trimmed upper edges. 6 5-year-old girl, *c.* 1869. Silk taffeta dress, low neckline filled with lace-edged blouse, fitted bodice with large velvet-edged pointed sham collar with tassel trim under wide frilled neckline, velvet detail repeated above flared cuffs of long sleeves, looped trailing ends from back of waistband and trim above pleated hemline on box-pleated skirt. Small felt hat with curled brim and shallow crown trimmed with ribbon band and trailing ends. Cloth boots with leather soles, heel backs, heels and pointed toecaps. 7 9-year-old girl, *c.* 1868. Collarless velvet cape with edge-to-edge hook fastening, ruched silk trimming between rows of contrast-colour silk piping, matching rosettes on edges of sloping shoulder seams, outside edges decorated with points of stiffened silk in contrasting colours. Striped silk dress, high neckline edged with pleated frill, long sleeves with narrow cuffs and full skirt. Small stiffened felt hat with curled brim and shallow crown with ribbon band and trailing ends, rosette and feather trim. Kid gloves. Knitted cotton stockings. Long cloth boots with leather soles, small heels, pointed toecaps and bound edges.

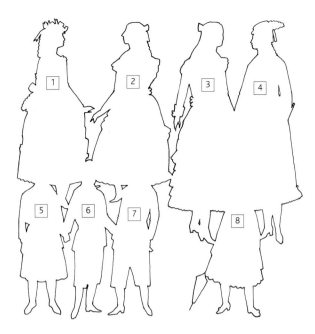

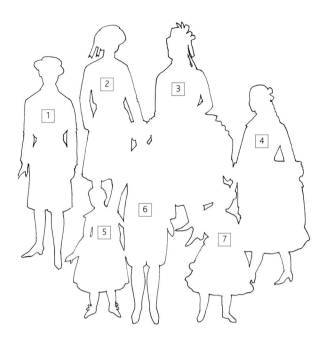

1870–1872

1 7-year-old girl, *c.* 1870. Silk taffeta dress, long sleeves with sewn cuffs, fitted bodice, high neckline with shallow stand collar, deep yoke seam, front and back, trimmed with self-fabric pleating, matching edges of split peplum and hemline of ruched overskirt, waist-sash with bow trim at back, decoration repeated on side seams, self-fabric knife-pleated underskirt. Tiny hat, worn tilted forward on head, with narrow brim and shallow crown decorated with ribbons and wax berries. Silk stockings. Short Short leather boots with side-button fastenings. 2 7-year-old girl, *c.* 1870. Silk dress, long sleeves with velvet ribbon trim on hems, matching shallow stand collar, yoke seams on fitted bodice, waist-belt with rosette above small bustle, overskirt and hemline of mid-calf-length skirt, edges, hems and detail decorated with frills of spotted cotton voile. Ribbon bow worn in hair. Silk stockings. Ankle-length leather boots with button fastenings and pointed toecaps. 3 12-year-old girl, *c.* 1872. Silk taffeta dress, long sleeves with deep cuffs trimmed with self-fabric rosette and pleating, fitted bodice centre front trimmed with row of covered buttons from under high neckline to top of wide waist-sash, shallow stand collar with pleated edge, panel seams from shoulder to waist trimmed with wide frills, cut with scalloped pinked edges, matching frills on open overskirt and four tiers above hemline of mid-calf-length skirt. Ribbon bow worn in hair at back. Silk stockings. Short leather boots with button fastenings and low stacked heels. 4 12-year-old girl, *c.* 1871. Hip-length edge-to-edge velvet jacket fastening at collarless neckline with small brooch, long sleeves gathered into narrow cuffs. Cotton blouse with lace-edged stand collar. Mid-calf-length patterned silk skirt with frilled hemline, cut with pointed pinked edges, skirt worn with wide ribbon belt decorated with buckle on front and back fastening. Straw hat worn tilted forward on head, narrow curled brim, shallow crown trimmed with velvet ribbon and large feather. Short cloth gloves. Long-handled parasol. Silk stockings. Long cloth boots with leather soles, side-button fastenings, square toecaps and low stacked heels. 5 4-year-old boy, *c.* 1871. Waist-length wool jacket, collarless, edge-to-edge and with long sleeves, edges trimmed with wool braid, matching hip-length waistcoat with centre-front hooked fastening and decorative double-breasted row of brass buttons, waistcoat worn with leather belt. Cotton shirt with large collar, worn with silk bow tie. Knee-length wool plaid kilt. Long socks. Cloth gaiters worn over leather slippers. 6 4-year-old boy, *c.* 1871. Wool suit: collarless hip-length jacket with buttoned strap fastening, buttoned belt, hip-level patch pockets, single breast pocket and long sleeves, edges and detail trimmed with wool braid, matching knee-length trousers. Cotton shirt with large collar, worn with narrow ribbon bow tie. Knitted cotton socks turned down over tops of leather boots with front laced fastenings, round toecaps and low stacked heels. 7 4-year-old boy, *c.* 1872. Cotton suit: waist-length jacket with buttoned strap fastening from under large collar to above inset buttoned waist-belt, long sleeves trimmed above wrists with narrow braid, edges and detail matching knee-length trousers. Brimless felt hat with bird's-wing decoration on one side. Cotton stockings. Ankle-length leather boots with elasticated side-gussets, pointed toecaps and stacked heels. 8 3-year-old girl, *c.* 1871. Single-breasted wool coat, large collar with scalloped edge, repeated on hems of flared sleeves, coat and skirt in matching fabric. Straw hat with narrow brim and tall crown trimmed with satin ribbons. Short cloth gloves. Long-handled parasol. Cotton stockings. Leather slippers with buttoned bar straps, low heels and rosette trim above round toes.

1873–1874

1 7-year-old boy, *c.* 1873. Waist-length linen jacket with buttoned strap fastening from under Peter Pan collar to above waist-level buckled belt, long sleeves with decorative braid trim above hems, matching patch pocket, hems of knee-length trousers and all other edges and detail. Stiffened straw hat with straight brim, shallow flat-topped crown with ribbon band and side bow trim. Short cloth gloves. Striped knitted cotton stockings. Cloth boots with leather soles, square toecaps and stacked heels. 2 10-year-old boy, *c.* 1873. Waist-length cotton jacket with buttoned strap fastening from under bow trim on large sailor collar to above waist-level buttoned waistband, long sleeves gathered into cuffs trimmed with coloured ribbon, matching hems and side seams of knee-length trousers and all other edges and detail. Collarless single-breasted cotton waistcoat. Cotton shirt with small collar and silk ribbon tie. Short cloth gloves. Coloured knitted cotton stockings. Ankle-length leather boots. 3 12-year-old girl, *c.* 1873. Double-breasted wool jacket with contrast-colour velvet collar and revers, sleeve cuffs on long sleeves, buttons and bindings. Knee-length checked wool pleated skirt with draped and buttoned plain wool overskirt, trimmed with checked wool and edged with points of stiffened plain wool. Cotton blouse with wing collar and long sleeves, worn with spotted ribbon tie. Small hat with turned-back brim, tall flat-topped crown and looped trim, all in fabric matching skirt, with velvet ribbon band and bow with trailing ends at back, feather trim. Short cloth gloves. Striped knitted cotton stockings. Leather boots with shaped tops, button fastenings, pointed toes and low stacked heels. 4 5-year-old girl, *c.* 1874. Short double-breasted wool coat with looped bustle at back, large collar trimmed with velvet, matching button fastenings and trim, detail above hemline, frilled cuffs on long sleeves. Knee-length cotton dress, small collar with frilled edge, matching two frills above hem. Ribbon bow worn in hair. Short cloth gloves. Striped knitted cotton stockings. Short cloth boots with elasticated side-gussets, leather soles, square toecaps and stacked heels. 5 18-month-old boy, *c.* 1874. Knee-length cotton frock, front-buttoned strap fastening trimmed with ribbon and embroidered lace, matching low square neckline and short cap sleeves, ribbon trim repeated on high waistband and in rows above hemline. Knitted cotton stockings. Cloth boots with ribbon bow-tie fastenings. 6 6-year-old boy, *c.* 1873. Collarless double-breasted wool jacket, edges braided in contrast colour, repeated above pointed sewn cuffs on long sleeves. Knee-length breeches in matching fabric. Cotton shirt with long sleeves and turned-down collar, worn with ribbon tie. Straw hat with curled brim, shallow crown trimmed with ribbon band and ostrich feather trim. Striped knitted cotton stockings. Leather slippers with buttoned bar straps and rosette trim above round toes. 7 3-year-old girl, *c.* 1874. Velvet coat, edge-to-edge hooked front fastening edged with swansdown, matching two-tier hemlines, hems of long sleeves and front edge of close-fitting bonnet with ribbon tie. Silk skirt with frilled hem detail. Short cloth gloves. Leather pumps with round toes and low heels worn with knee-length cloth gaiters, side-button fastenings and stirrups under foot.

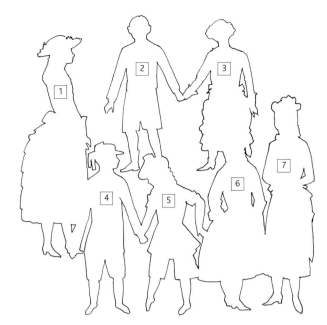

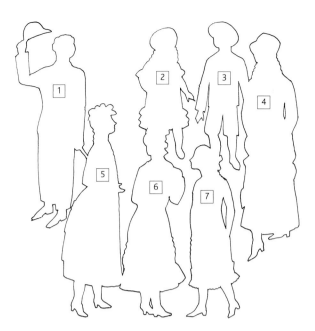

1875–1877

1 7-year-old girl, *c.* 1875. Cotton dress with fitted bodice, front button fastening with contrast-colour covered buttons, matching stand collar with frilled edge, repeated on full-length sleeve cuffs and as large bow on back waist above frill-edged peplum, mid-calf-length plain skirt with five tiers of frills at back. Straw hat with wide brim trimmed with rows of frills and posies of silk flowers, shallow crown with ribbon band. Short cloth gloves. Knitted cotton stockings. Cloth boots with side-button fastenings, leather soles, toecaps and stacked heels.
2 3-year-old boy, *c.* 1877. Two-piece wool suit: double-breasted waist-length jacket with pearl buttons matching trim on long sleeves under sewn cuffs and on side seams of knee-length trousers, braid-trimmed edges and detail. Cotton shirt with large collar and long sleeves. Short knitted cotton socks. Ankle-length leather boots with elasticated side-gussets, shiny toecaps and stacked heels.
3 3-year-old girl, *c.* 1877. Cotton satin dress, long fitted bodice with buttoned strap fastening, long sleeves, deep cuffs trimmed with contrast-colour frilled edges, matching frilled edge of Peter Pan collar, bow trim at neck, waist front and back and tiers of deep frills on draped skirt. Coloured knitted cotton stockings. Ankle-length leather boots with elasticated side-gussets, shiny toecaps and low heels.
4 5-year-old boy, *c.* 1875. Two-piece wool suit: double-breasted hip-length jacket with brass buttons, stand collar and wide revers with braid-trimmed edges, matching sewn cuffs on long sleeves and hip-level pockets; breeches buttoned on knee. Stiffened straw boater with shallow crown trimmed with ribbon band and bow and trailing ends at back. Striped knitted cotton stockings. Long leather boots with round toes and stacked heels.
5 3-year-old girl, *c.* 1876. Cotton bathing suit: collarless hip-length top, hooked front fastening decorated with contrast-colour looped bows, matching trim on short sleeves and side seams of knee-length shorts, edges and detail also bound in contrast colour. Straw hat with wide stiffened brim trimmed with loops of ribbon, tiny topless crown. Long rubberized cotton heelless boots, fastening with four buttoned bar straps, rosette trim above round toes.
6 5-year-old girl, *c.* 1876. Silk dress with hip-length fitted bodice, three-quarter-length sleeves with button trim above contrast-colour cuffs, matching double-breasted button trim on back panel of bodice, contrast colour repeated in wide binding on bodice hem, low sash and fringed bow at back of mid-calf-length skirt and sham apron at front. Straw hat with wide brim and tall crown, decorated with velvet ribbon band and bow, silk flowers and ostrich feathers.
7 8-year-old girl, *c.* 1877. Cotton dress with fitted bodice, edge-to-edge front hook fastening, trimmed with large contrast-colour bows from under high stand collar with frilled edge to above pleated hemline of draped skirt, repeated on long sleeves above pleated cuffs and at low waist level at back, mid-calf-length tiered pleated skirt. Straw hat with curled brim, low rounded crown, looped ribbon at back with trailing ends, silk flowers inside and outside brim. Short cloth gloves. Leather shoes with pointed toes and high heels, cloth uppers with side-button fastenings.

1878–1879

1 9-year-old boy, *c.* 1878. Single-breasted hip-length wool jacket with high single-button fastening, narrow collar and revers with braided edges, matching stitched cuffs on long sleeves, flap pockets and rounded cut-away fronts. Collarless single-breasted velvet waistcoat. Cotton shirt with long sleeves and large collar, worn with large silk bow tie. Ankle-length straight-cut wool trousers. Bowler hat with curled brim and high rounded crown with wide band. Walking stick with silver handle. Ankle-length leather boots with elasticated side-gussets, round toes and low stacked heels.
2 2-year-old girl, *c.* 1879. Unfitted cotton dress with low square neckline edged with embroidered braids, matching hems of short sleeves above wide frill, panels on each side of centre-front decorative button trim and at hip level above three tiers of frills. Dress worn with collarless cotton blouse. Straw hat, wide up-swept brim with bound edge, crown trimmed with silk flowers. Long socks. Leather shoes, T-straps with button fastenings.
3 3-year-old boy, *c.* 1878. Striped wool suit: unfitted double-breasted jacket with narrow collar and revers, long sleeves and patch pockets, top-stitched edges and detail; knee breeches in matching fabric. Cotton shirt with long sleeves and large collar, worn with large silk bow tie. Straw hat, up-swept brim with bound edge, matching band on rounded crown and trailing ends at back. Long ribbed wool socks turned down over cloth gaiters with stirrups under feet of leather shoes.
4 10-year-old girl, *c.* 1879. Hip-length wool tweed jacket with fitted bodice over hips, edge-to-edge hooked fastening trimmed with fur, matching collar, cuffs on long sleeves, two mid-calf-length pointed panels below jacket hem at front and large hand muff. Ankle-length wool skirt with pleated detail around hemline. Felt hat with narrow brim and tall crown trimmed with ribbon band and bow. Leather gloves. Knitted wool stockings. Leather boots with side-button fastenings, pointed toes and high stacked heels.
5 8-year-old girl, *c.* 1878. Mid-calf-length silk dress, long fitted bodice with wide ruched panel at front from under stand collar to above pleated hemline of underskirt, pleated detail repeated on back hem edge of draped overskirt, sleeve cuffs on long sleeves and edge of collar. Hat covered in dress fabric, curled brim and low crown trimmed with pleated self-fabric. Short cloth gloves. Long boots, cloth uppers with side-button fastenings, leather fronts, heel backs and stacked heels.
6 5-year-old girl, *c.* 1878. Silk dress with long fitted bodice, back panel seams from shoulder to hip level with inset decorative buttoned tabs, matching detail above deep cuffs on long sleeves, skirt ruched in panels above gathered frill hemline. Straw hat with narrow brim, tall crown trimmed with loops of ribbon and silk flowers. Large silk ribbon bow worn in hair at back. Knitted silk stockings. Leather shoes with low-cut fronts, pointed toes and stacked heels.
7 5-year-old girl, *c.* 1878. Silk dress with long fitted bodice, low square neckline bound with contrast-colour edge, matching hems of short sleeves, hip-level front panel, turned-back revers with button detail on either side of draped front panel of skirt and band with pleated edges above hemline. Large silk ribbon bow worn in hair at back. Coral bead necklace. Knitted silk stockings. Long cloth gaiters with side-button fastenings and stirrups under feet of leather shoes with pointed toes and stacked heels.

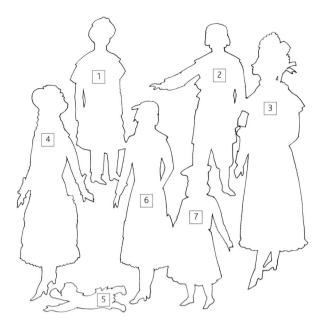

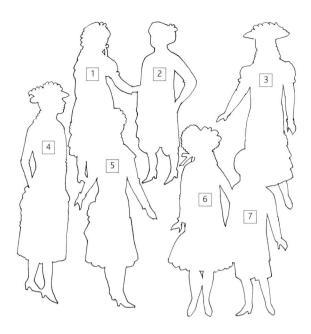

1880 – 1881

1 4-year-old boy, *c.* 1881. Single-breasted wool overcoat, buttoning from under shoulder-wide double-cape collar to hem of knee-length skirts, long sleeves, deep cuffs with button detail, repeated on low hip-level patch pockets set onto side flaps, top-stitched edges and detail, coat worn with buckled leather belt on low hipline. Cotton shirt with stand collar and long sleeves. Ankle-length wool trousers. Felt hat with turned-back brim, high crown and pompon trim. Cloth spats with side-button fastenings worn over leather shoes with stacked heels. 2 4-year-old boy, *c.* 1880. Striped linen sailor suit: long single-breasted jacket, fastening from under shoulder-wide collar trimmed with contrast-colour band, matching cuffs on long sleeves, tops of four patch pockets, buttons and outsized bow tie, jacket worn with buckled leather belt on low hipline; knee breeches; high-neck under-vest in jacket fabric. Striped knitted cotton socks. Cloth boots with side-button fastenings, leather soles, heels and pointed toecaps. 3 10-year-old girl, *c.* 1881. Wool coat with double-breasted fastening from under pleated cape collar to above hemline of mid-calf-length skirts, long sleeves, deep cuffs with pleated edges and button trim, button detail repeated on low hip-level pockets, pleats repeated from hip level on side and back panels of skirts, coat worn over cotton dress with frilled hemline. Straw hat with tall crown trimmed with ribbon band and bow at back, wide brim decorated with ostrich feathers. Short cloth gloves. Long kid boots with side-button fastenings, square toes and high stacked heels. 4 8-year-old girl, *c.* 1881. Silk dress with fitted hip-level bodice, high round neckline with ruffled edge in contrast colour, matching cuffs on long sleeves, ends hanging to hip level, scarf-effect above pin-tucked yoke, side panel seams trimmed with fancy lace, matching detail between pleats of tiered skirt, self-fabric swagged overskirt with gathered and pleated hanging panels. Hat covered in silk to match dress, wide brim and tall crown with looped ribbon rosette trimming. Coloured knitted silk stockings. Long kid boots with side-button fastenings, buttons, high heels and square toecaps in contrast colour. 5 1-year-old girl, *c.* 1880. Silk dress cut in one piece with no waist seam, large lace collar threaded with silk ribbon, matching deep cuffs on long sleeves, hemline of flared skirt and inset back panel with large bow. Knitted cotton socks. Cloth boots with side-button fastenings. 6 8-year-old girl, *c.* 1880. Silk dress cut in panels with no waist seam, large lace collar, matching edges of deep cuffs on long sleeves, low hip-level pocket, detail on edge of hemline and above hemline of mid-calf-length skirt, outsized contrast-colour bow set into panel seams at low hip level at back. Silk ribbon bow worn in hair at back. Long kid boots with side-button fastenings, pointed toes and high heels. 7 4-year-old girl, *c.* 1880. Plain cotton dress, bloused bodice with striped cotton sailor collar, matching high-neck under-vest, lower part of long sleeves to elbow level and panel above hemline of contrast-colour gathered skirt, contrast colour repeated as bow tie and bindings of high neck and sleeve hems. Knitted beret with pompon trim on top. Long leather boots with side-button fastenings, patent leather toecaps and low stacked heels.

1882 – 1883

1 5-year-old girl, *c.* 1882. Silk dress, long fitted bodice cut without waist seam, shoulder-wide lace collar above short puff oversleeves, matching cuffs on long sleeves, floating back panel caught at waist level by smocked half-belt and at low hip level by wide contrast-colour sash tied into outsized bow, mid-calf-length skirt with frilled hemline. Silk-covered bonnet with narrow brim and shallow crown, draped in self-fabric and trimmed with ribbons and silk flowers, bow tie under chin. Knitted silk stockings. Leather boots with stacked heels. 2 4-year-old boy, *c.* 1882. Wool suit: knee-length single-breasted coat, fastening with contrast-colour velvet-covered buttons, matching collar and revers, fancy cuffs on long sleeves, trim on hip-level patch pockets and turned-back front facings of skirts; knee breeches to match coat. Cotton shirt worn with silk tie and tiepin. Straw hat with turned-back brim, edge bound with ribbon, matching rosette on one side. Knitted stockings. Leather boots with side-button fastenings, pointed toes and stacked heels. 3 5-year-old girl, *c.* 1882. Cotton dress with long fitted bodice, cut in one without waist seam, lace collar and cuffs, contrast-colour and patterned puff sleeves, matching inset trim on long sleeves, gathered and smocked front panel and draped sash above frilled three-tier skirt. Straw hat with wide brim and shallow crown covered with ostrich feathers. Short cloth gloves. Coloured knitted cotton stockings. Leather boots with side-button fastenings and pointed toes. 4 10-year-old girl, *c.* 1883. Silk dress, long fitted bodice cut without waist seam, waist-length contrast-colour inset panel with self-fabric covered button trim and coloured piping, matching small stand collar with asymmetric bow trim, cuffs on long sleeves and rosette on one side of draped overskirt, pleated underskirt to match front bodice, cotton frill at neck and wrists. Straw hat with wide brim and shallow crown covered with ostrich feathers. Short cloth gloves. Long cloth gaiters with side-button fastenings and stirrups; leather boots with pointed toes and high heels. 5 8-year-old girl, *c.* 1882. Knee-length velvet coat, bodice and skirt cut in panels without waist seam, shoulder-wide cape with lace collar and trimming, matching cuffs on long sleeves, hip-level patch pockets and hem of skirts, outsized satin bow threaded through fancy buckle on hip level at back above box pleats. Cloth hat with pleated brim and shallow crown, wide ribbon and ostrich feather trim. Short kid gloves. Knitted wool stockings. Long leather boots with side-button fastenings and high heels. 6 7-year-old girl, *c.* 1883. Cotton dress, straight hip-length bodice with gathered front panel from smocking under large collar to above wide bow-tied hip-level belt, matching bow tie at neck and binding on hems of long sleeves, knee-length gathered skirt, cotton frill at neck and wrists. Lace-trimmed petticoat. Cotton bonnet with pleated brim and gathered crown trimmed with silk flowers, bow tie under chin. Knitted cotton stockings. Long leather boots with side-button fastenings and pointed toes. 7 5-year-old boy, *c.* 1882. Linen suit: hip-length double-breasted jacket with velvet shawl collar, matching edges of jacket, low-slung belt and binding and trim on long sleeves; short trousers in matching fabric. Cotton shirt with frilled collar and cuffs, worn with silk bow tie. Straw hat with turned-back brim. Striped knitted cotton stockings. Long leather boots with side-button fastenings, pointed toes and stacked heels.

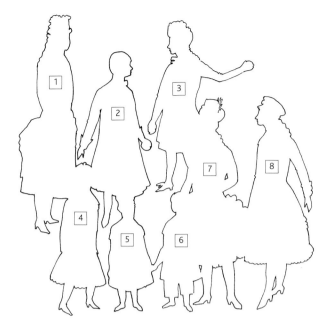

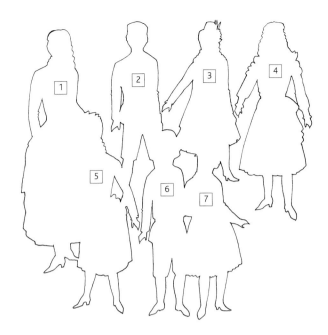

1884–1885

1 6-year-old girl, *c.* 1884. Silk dress, gathered front bodice, pleated overskirt, low neckline edged with contrast colour, matching deep cuffs on long sleeves, waistband, swathed apron front, bustle and underskirt, low neckline filled with mock blouse, lace-edged stand collar, matching lace frill under sleeve cuffs. Straw hat, edge of narrow brim turned back, tall crown, ribbon band, ostrich feather trim. Coloured cotton stockings. Cloth boots with side-button fastenings, leather soles, pointed fronts and stacked heels. 2 4-year-old boy, *c.* 1884. Three-piece wool suit: edge-to-edge long jacket with large lace-edged collar worn with outsized silk bow tie, matching lace-edged cuffs on long sleeves, large patch and button-trimmed flap pockets; single-breasted long waistcoat above pleated skirt. Wool stockings. Cloth boots with side-button fastenings and pointed leather fronts. 3 4-year-old girl, *c.* 1885. Three-piece silk suit: edge-to-edge long jacket with shoulder-wide collar, looped ribbon bow fastening, long sleeves with frilled hems, large patch pockets with button trim; unfitted dress with diagonal tucks either side of mock strap fastening with button trim, hip-level inset belt above short flared skirt with off-centre split, pleated underskirt, top-stitched edges and detail. Felt hat, front brim turned back, tall crown with band and bow, ostrich feather trim. Coloured wool stockings. Leather shoes with ribbon fastenings, pointed toes and stacked heels. 4 4-year-old girl, *c.* 1884. Striped cotton dress with high round neckline, long unfitted bodice with horizontal contrast-colour cotton satin inset bands, set between vertical bands in same colour, matching covered buttons, edges of cuffs on long sleeves and hip-belt above knee-length panelled skirt, wide lace-edged collar, lace repeated set into waist seam, under cuffs and on mid seam and hem of skirt. Large ribbon bow worn in hair at back. Coloured cotton stockings. Long cloth spats with side-button fastenings and stirrups, worn above leather shoes with pointed toes and stacked heels. 5 2-year-old boy, *c.* 1884. Knee-length single-breasted cotton bathing dress, low neckline embroidered with anchors and edged with fancy braid, matching edges of short sleeves, hemline and strap and button fastenings set between panels of cotton lace. Cotton peaked cap, gathered crown with bow trim on front. Heelless cloth bathing shoes with buttoned bar straps. 6 2-year-old girl, *c.* 1885. Two-piece cotton bathing suit: hip-length single-breasted jacket with double collar, short sleeves, front opening, buttoned waist-belt and hem of gathered skirts edged with fancy braid, matching hems of short trousers. Turban. Heelless cloth shoes with ribbon ties. 7 8-year-old girl, *c.* 1885. Velvet dress with fitted hip-length bodice, high stand collar in contrast colour with bow trim and frilled cotton edge, matching frills below hems of sewn cuffs on long sleeves, puffs on central panel above bow trim at waist level, contrast-colour velvet repeated on pleated side panels and bustle, hemline trimmed with mock petticoat frill of lace. Straw hat, narrow brim with bound edge, tall crown draped and looped with silk ribbon and trimmed with tiny feathers. Coloured cotton stockings. Long cloth spats with stirrups, leather shoes with pointed toes and stacked heels. 8 9-year-old girl, *c.* 1885. Velvet dress with long fitted bodice and flared skirt cut in one piece without waist seam, large collar trimmed with braid and edged with lace, matching buttoned cuffs on long sleeves, buttoned flap pockets, small bustle and centre-front panel, lace trim on vertical panel seams and on edge of hemline above mock petticoat frills. Cloth hat with frilled brim and gathered crown above velvet ribbon band and bow. Ribbed wool stockings. High leather boots with side-button fastenings, pointed toes and stacked heels.

1886–1887

1 12-year-old girl, *c.* 1886. Checked silk dress with fitted cross-over bodice forming low neckline, edges trimmed with buttons, contrast-colour in-fill, high stand collar with frilled edge and button trim, matching cuffs on long sleeves and detail above tucks on hemline of contrast-colour underskirt, draped apron-effect overskirt and back bustle in checked silk. Long leather boots with side-button fastenings, pointed toes and high heels. 2 6-year-old boy, *c.* 1886. Two-piece wool tweed suit: long single-breasted jacket with narrow collar and revers, long sleeves with sewn cuffs and button trim, pleats from shoulder to hemline, held in place by buttoned waist-belt, top-stitched edges and detail; knee-length trousers. Cotton shirt with stiffened stand collar and cuffs, worn with silk scarf. Brimless wool tweed hat with high crown. Knitted wool stockings. Long leather boots. 3 4-year-old girl, *c.* 1887. Three-piece cotton suit: long edge-to-edge jacket, hook fastening under stand collar with braid trimming, matching sewn cuffs on long sleeves and jacket edges; waistcoat with diagonal pleats and button fastening; box-pleated skirt. Cotton blouse, stand collar with frilled edge, matching sleeve cuffs. Straw hat, wide brim turned up at front and trimmed with silk flowers, matching decoration with feathers on one side of tall flat-topped crown. Ribbed knitted wool stockings. Leather boots with pointed toes and stacked heels. 4 7-year-old girl, *c.* 1887. Cotton dress with fitted bodice, low V-shaped neckline with ruched edge, machine-made frilled lace trim and machine-embroidered lace in-fill with pleated edge, lace frills repeated on shoulder epaulettes and above hemline of gathered skirt, embroidery and pleating repeated on cuffs of long full sleeves, wide contrast-colour sash above smocked hip yoke, tied into bow at back. Dark knitted cotton stockings. Leather boots with shaped tops, pointed toes and high heels. 5 6-year-old girl, *c.* 1886. Striped glazed cotton dress, fitted bodice with contrast-colour waistcoat-effect single-breasted fastening from under stand collar with frilled edge to pointed hemline, frills repeated below button-trimmed plain fabric cuffs of long sleeves, bands of plain colour with tassel trim on either side of waistcoat, matching fabric of draped bustle at back, striped skirt with unpressed pleats. Dyed straw hat with wide turned-back brim, ostrich feather trimming. Dark knitted cotton stockings. Leather boots with pointed toes, high heels and cloth uppers. 6 5-year-old boy, *c.* 1887. Two-piece linen suit: long jacket with buttoned strap fastening from under large stiffened cotton shirt collar to hemline, matching cuffs, two chest-level flap pockets, long sleeves with cuffs, jacket worn with narrow leather buckled belt, silk scarf knotted under shirt collar; breeches gathered into bands at knee level. Straw hat with narrow brim and large crown, striped band with bow at back and trailing ends. Striped knitted cotton socks. Leather shoes with bar straps and low heels. 7 4-year-old girl, *c.* 1886. Silk dress with long bodice gathered above tied knot at hip level on centre front, high neckline with pleated edge, repeated under sleeve cuffs, neck edge bound in dark colour, matching edges of square collar, cuffs on long sleeves, fringed hip-level flaps and petal-shaped panels above contrast-colour pleated skirt. Straw hat, wide brim turned up on either side and bound with silk, crown covered with looped striped silk ribbon. Long cloth spats with side-button fastenings and stirrups under leather shoes with pointed toes and high heels.

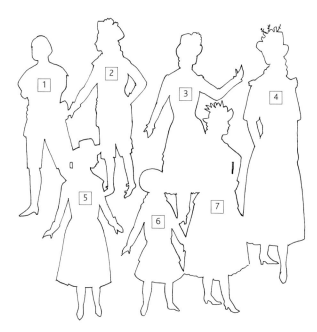

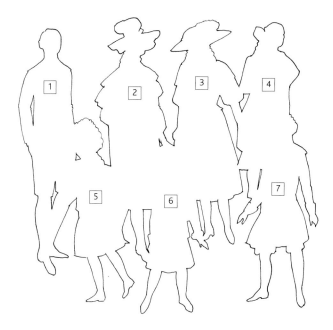

1888 –1889

1 6-year-old boy, *c.* 1889. Silk satin two-piece suit: hip-length single-breasted jacket, fastening with outsized buttons, shoulder-wide lace collar, matching cuffs on long sleeves, knee-length trousers, contrast-colour silk satin sash with fringed edges, tied in large bow on side hip. Striped cotton stockings. Long leather boots with pointed toes and stacked heels.
2 5-year-old boy, *c.* 1889. Striped velvet two-piece suit: hip-length single-breasted jacket, fastening from under shoulder-wide lace-edged collar to hem, matching edges of deep plain cotton cuffs on long sleeves, knee-length trousers, wide silk sash with tasselled ends, tied on side hip. Straw hat with wide turned-back brim, tall crown trimmed with ostrich feathers. Striped cotton stockings. Heelless leather slippers with bow trim on centre front and on fronts of bar straps. 3 7-year-old girl, *c.* 1888. Striped silk two-piece suit: jacket with long fitted bodice, stand collar trimmed with velvet, matching cuffs on long sleeves, hemline and two bows trimming bustle, darker self-colour pleating on all edges, hems and detail. Straw hat with wide brim and tall flat-topped crown draped with silk, posy of silk flowers set on front. Silk ribbon bow in hair at back. Short kid gloves. Striped cotton stockings. Long leather boots with side-button fastenings and stacked heels. 4 12-year-old girl, *c.* 1889. Cotton dress with fitted bodice, shoulder-wide neckline filled with fine cotton sham blouse, frilled lace edging and lace-trimmed stand collar, matching inset bands on fitted lower part of full sleeves and three bands set into full mid-calf-length skirt, wide cotton satin waist-sash tied into outsized bow on side. Straw hat with narrow brim turned up at front and back, flat-topped crown with velvet band, ruched ribbon and spray of silk leaves front trim. Short kid gloves. Long suede boots with side-button fastenings, leather pointed toecaps, heel backs and stacked heels.
5 4-year-old girl, *c.* 1889. Cotton velvet knee-length coat with fitted bodice, open front hooked to waistband of dress, front edges and wide lace revers bordered with lace, matching cuffs of long sleeves, cut-away skirts, muslin dress, gathered front bodice with contrast-colour draped velvet stand collar, matching pleated waistband, full gathered skirt. Straw hat with wide turned-back brim, edge bound with velvet, matching wide band around tall crown and trailing ends at back. Short cloth gloves. Cotton stockings. Leather boots with shaped tops and pointed toes. 6 2-year-old boy, *c.* 1888. Hip-length velvet jacket, shawl collar edged with braid, matching cuffs on long sleeves, hip-level belt with clasp fastening and edges of open panelled skirt. Striped silk dress with gathered bodice from under draped velvet stand collar, knee-length box-pleated skirt. Straw hat with large brim, worn on back of head. Knee-length wool socks. Leather shoes with buttoned bar straps, round toes and low heels. 7 8-year-old girl, *c.* 1888. Edge-to-edge cloth jacket with hook fastening under wide revers, long sleeves with velvet-trimmed cuffs, matching all edges. Long single-breasted embroidered silk waistcoat with wide revers and button-trimmed flap pockets. Muslin blouse with gathered front under velvet stand collar. Pleated cloth skirt. Straw hat with brim turned up at front, edged with striped fabric, matching band around shallow crown, exotic bird trim set at front. Short kid gloves. Striped cotton stockings. Cloth ankle-length boots with side-button fastenings, leather heel backs, pointed toes and high heels.

1890 –1891

1 10-year-old boy, *c.* 1890. Wool tweed suit: single-breasted jacket with high collar and revers, long sleeves with button trim, single breast patch pocket and two matching pockets at hip level; knee-length trousers. Cotton shirt with shoulder-wide collar, worn with large silk bow tie. Long ribbed wool stockings. Ankle-length leather boots with laced and hooked front fastenings, pointed toecaps and low stacked heels. 2 8-year-old girl, *c.* 1891. Unfitted wool tweed coat with single-breasted button fastening through two-tier cape collar to knee level in mid-calf-length skirts, long full sleeves gathered into cuffs, front panel seams, hems and edges bound in contrast colour. Cotton hat with wide unstructured brim and small gathered unstructured crown trimmed with contrast-colour ribbon and bow. Short kid gloves. Coloured stockings. Long leather boots with laced and hooked front fastenings, pointed toecaps and low stacked heels. 3 8-year-old girl, *c.* 1890. Silk bridesmaid's dress, fitted bodice with tucks on either side of centre front under jacket-effect side panels, full sleeves gathered into elbow-length lace-trimmed cuffs, matching trim on mid-calf-length gathered skirt, large lace collar matching apron-effect on front of skirt, trimmed from underneath with velvet ribbon loops and ends, matching decoration on shoulders. Large silk-covered hat with wide brim, shallow draped crown, large ostrich feather trim. Long silk stockings. Kid shoes with buttoned bar straps, pointed toes and high heels. 4 5-year-old girl, *c.* 1891. Collarless cotton overdress, smocking under high yoke seam, above-knee-length skirt and full sleeves gathered into deep cuffs. Cotton underdress with ribbon-trimmed collar, matching sleeve cuffs and hemline of knee-length skirt. Large ribbon worn at back of head. Long knitted cotton stockings. Leather shoes with low stacked heels. 5 4-year-old girl, *c.* 1890. Single-breasted wool coat with outsized self-fabric covered button fastening from under shoulder-wide collar with contrast-colour scallop-edged overcollar, matching cuffs on long sleeves and hemline of knee-length skirts, self-fabric belt with round covered buckle and button fastening. Large silk-covered bonnet, trimmed with silk pleating, silk rosettes and ostrich feathers and ribbons tied into a bow under chin. Short cloth gloves. Long knitted cotton stockings. Leather shoes with buttoned bar straps, pointed toes and low stacked heels. 6 2-year-old boy, *c.* 1891. Velvet suit: short edge-to-edge bolero jacket with rounded edges and long sleeves, matching knee-length gathered skirt. Cotton shirt, shoulder-wide collar with frilled lace edge, matching centre front and sleeve cuffs, worn with large silk bow tie at neck. Long knitted cotton stockings. Cloth spats, stirrups under leather shoes with pointed toes and low stacked heels. 7 5-year-old boy, *c.* 1890. Knee-length striped cotton dress with single-breasted button fastening from under shoulder-wide lace collar, matching cuffs on long sleeves, full skirts and hip-level belt with round buckle, dress worn with ribbon bow tie at neck. Lace knickers. Striped knitted cotton stockings. Leather boots with front-laced and hooked front fastenings, square toecaps and low stacked heels.

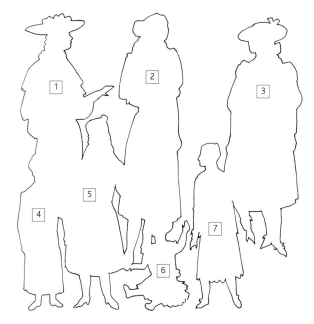

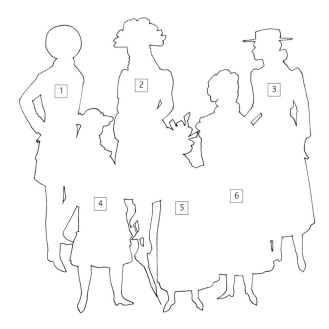

1892 –1894

1 8-year-old girl, c. 1894. Silk bridesmaid's dress, bloused bodice with smocked stand collar bound with contrast-colour matching vertical inset bands and horizontal band at chest level, trimmed with two rosettes, cuffs on full sleeves with rosette trim repeated at elbow level, contrast-colour waist-sash above gathered skirt, dress worn with lace shoulder cape. Silk-covered hat with wide unstructured wavy brim and tiny crown covered with an outsized looped bow in contrast colour. Vertically striped knitted silk stockings. Silk-covered shoes with high heels. 2 10-year-old girl, c. 1893. Fine wool dress with bloused bodice, smocked yoke with frilled edges, frilled stand collar, matching cuffs on long sleeves, inset waistband, frilled epaulettes and frills on elbow-length upper sleeves, knee-length gathered skirt. Large ribbon bow worn in hair at back. Knitted wool stockings. Long leather boots with hooked and laced front fastenings, pointed toes and high heels. 3 7-year-old girl, c. 1892. Unfitted wool tweed coat, single-breasted fastening with outsized self-fabric covered buttons under narrow collar and revers, gathered upper sleeves above tight-fitting elbow-length cuffs, braid-trimmed edges and detail. Straw hat with wide stiffened brim and shallow flat-topped crown with ribbon band, bow trim and wired ends at back. Short kid gloves. Knitted wool stockings. Leather shoes with ribbon laces, pointed toes and high heels. 4 2-year-old boy, c. 1893. Mid-calf-length linen frock, pleated bodice with concealed front fastening, large square collar trimmed with lace, matching cuffs on long sleeves and wide belt with concealed fastening, mid-calf-length box-pleated skirts. Brimless cloth hat with flat-topped crown gathered onto wide contrast-colour stiffened band. Cloth gaiters with side-button fastenings and stirrups under leather shoes with round toes and low heels. 5 5-year-old girl, c. 1894. Double-breasted wool coat with shoulder cape, large fur collar and matching hand muff, side slanting hip-level pockets in mid-calf-length flared skirts, top-stitched edges and detail. Brimless fur hat with small curled feather and brooch trim on one side, ribbon ties from either side fastened in bow under chin. Long leather boots with pointed toecaps and high heels. 6 10-month-old girl, c. 1892. Cotton muslin dress, fitted bodice with gathered front panel, low neckline with embroidered frill and trimmed with contrast-colour ruched silk ribbon, matching short sleeves and hem of full skirt, wide ribbon sash and rosette in matching silk with trailing ends. Cotton muslin bonnet with full gathered crown and pleated front edge trimmed with lace, large contrast-colour silk ribbon bow trim on front. Coral necklace. Knitted cotton socks. Heelless cloth boots with scalloped button fastenings. 7 3-year-old boy, c. 1892. Two-piece linen suit: double-breasted hip-length jacket with narrow lace-edged shawl collar, matching cuffs on long sleeves, hip-level flap pockets and hemlines of both jacket and mid-calf-length full skirt. Long knitted cotton stockings. Heelless leather shoes with bow-trimmed bar straps and tiny rosette trim above round toes.

1895 –1896

1 10-year-old boy, c. 1896. Short wool coat, double-breasted button fastening under wide collar and revers with braided edges, matching edges of deep cuffs on long sleeves, hip-level flap pockets, panel seams and hem. Cotton shirt with attached collar, worn with large spotted silk bow tie. Wool trousers with stirrups under feet. Straw hat, wide turned-back brim with bound edge. Leather gloves. Suede boots with patent leather heels and square toecaps. 2 9-year-old girl, c. 1895. Knee-length velvet coat, fitted bodice with soft pleats under shoulder-wide yoke, concealed front button fastening from under buttoned stand collar, full-length leg-of-mutton sleeves and full skirts. Large fur hand muff. Large cloth-covered hat with wide brim turned up at front and back, crown trimmed with ostrich feathers and looped ribbons. Knee-length cloth gaiters with side-button fastenings, worn over leather shoes with pointed toes. 3 12-year-old girl, c. 1896. Cotton blouse, bloused bodice with back fastening, gathers from under front yoke seam, trimmed with double row of self-fabric frills, gathers continuing under high stand collar, long full sleeves gathered into buttoned cuffs. Mid-calf-length fine wool skirt, cut in flared panels, worn with wide contrast-colour belt with fancy clasp fastening. Straw boater with narrow, stiffened brim and tall flat-topped crown with wide striped ribbon band. Large ribbon bow worn in hair at back. Long leather boots with hooked and laced front fastenings, pointed toes and low stacked heels. 4 6-year-old girl, c. 1896. Unfitted sleeveless cotton work-smock with back fastening, high neckline with frilled edge, matching edge of rounded yoke seam from shoulder to shoulder and detail above hem of short gathered skirt, smock worn over knee-length striped cotton dress, sleeves gathered from shoulder to elbow and tight to wrist level. Straw hat with unstructured double brim and shallow crown trimmed with ribbon band, artificial fruit and flowers. Striped knitted wool stockings. Long cloth boots with hooked and laced front fastenings, leather soles, heels and pointed toecaps. 5 4-year-old girl, c. 1896. Long checked wool coat, single-breasted fastening with outsized buttons from under velvet shawl collar, matching cuffs on long leg-of-mutton sleeves and diagonal hip-level pockets, mid-calf-length flared skirts with side slits, edges and detail bound with contrast-colour wool braid. Patterned cotton dress with ribbon-trimmed stand collar and cuffs. Cloth hat, turned-back brim with scalloped edge trimmed with ruched ribbon, crown decorated with wired striped ribbons. Short cloth gloves. Velvet reticule bag. Rolled umbrella with long handle. Leather boots with low heels, pointed toes and cloth uppers. 6 8-year-old girl, c. 1895. Mid-calf-length wool tweed coat, double-breasted button fastening under shoulder-wide cape edged with fur, matching collar and cuffs of long leg-of-mutton sleeves, diagonal hip-level flap pockets in flared skirts. Brimless velvet bonnet gathered onto wide embroidered ribbon band, matching ties fastening under chin in bow. Short leather gloves. Leather boots with pointed toes and low heels.

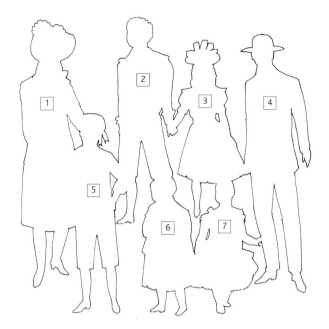

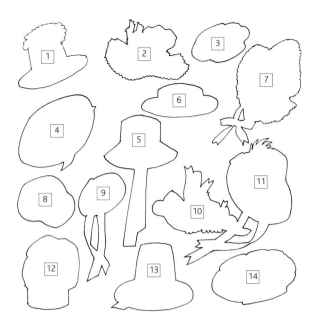

1897–1899

1 9-year-old girl, *c.* 1899. Fine wool suit: edge-to-edge hip-length jacket, held together at waist level with self-fabric buttoned strap, flared skirts with side vents, full-length sleeves, silk-faced revers, knee-length flared skirt, matching jacket fabric, top-stitched edges and detail. Checked silk taffeta blouse with high neck, ending in outsized bow tie at throat, centre-front buttoned strap fastening to low waist level, full-length sleeves. Felt hat with turned-back brim, trimmed with single checked silk taffeta rosette on side front, matching fan of pleats above crown, matching blouse fabric. Short kid gloves. Silk stockings. Leather shoes with high heels and buckle trim above pointed toes. 2 6-year-old boy, *c.* 1897. Plain cotton shirt with bloused bodice, centre-front buttoned strap fastening edged on either side with frilled lace, matching shoulder-wide collar and turned-back cuffs on long sleeves. Velvet breeches gathered into band at knee level. Striped cotton stockings. Leather shoes with laced fastenings, pointed toes and stacked heels. 3 3-year-old girl, *c.* 1898. Patterned cotton dress with box-pleated bodice under shoulder-wide yoke, plain cotton inset trim, matching stand collar, edges of stiffened epaulettes, band on pleated puff sleeves and buckled waist-belt, knee-length box-pleated skirt. Dyed straw boater with stiffened brim and flat-topped crown, trimmed with wired striped silk ribbon. Long cotton stockings. Short leather boots with side-button fastenings and pointed toes. 4 12-year-old boy, *c.* 1899. Single-breasted striped cotton hip-length jacket with high button fastening under narrow collar and revers, full-length sleeves with stitched cuffs, welted breast pocket, matching hip-level pockets. Collar-attached cotton shirt with buttoned strap fastening and long sleeves, worn with short striped silk necktie. Ankle-length wool flannel trousers with fly front, elasticated waist-belt with snake fastening. Fine straw hat with wide brim, turned up at sides, tall crown with centre-front crease and wide ribbon band. Two-tone lace-up shoes with pointed toecaps and low stacked heels. 5 7-year-old boy, *c.* 1899. Striped cotton sailor suit: bloused top with centre-front buttoned strap fastening under shoulder-wide plain cotton collar and contrast-colour bow tie, single breast patch pocket, long sleeves with buttoned cuffs; knee-length trousers with fly fronts; knitted cotton undershirt with high round neckline and small anchor embroidered on chest. Brimless sailor's hat, wide band trimmed with ribbon, trailing ends at back and contrast-colour flat-topped crown. Long cotton stockings. Leather shoes with buttoned bar straps, pointed toes and high heels. 6 2-year-old girl, *c.* 1897. Cotton sailor suit: edge-to-edge jacket with six large pearl button trim, long sleeves gathered into cuffs and shoulder-wide plain cotton collar; knee-length box-pleated skirt from wide waistband; striped knitted cotton undershirt with high round neckline. Brimless knitted cotton pull-on hat with contrast-colour inset band. Long cotton stockings. Long boots with hooked and laced front fastenings, round toes and low heels. 7 18-month-old girl, *c.* 1897. Cotton muslin dress with long horizontally pin-tucked bodice, matching frilled lace-trimmed gathered skirt, low V-shaped neckline with inserted frilled lace and filled with vertically pin-tucked panel to under high narrow lace-edged round neckline, short frilled lace sleeves, contrast-colour ribbon bow trim on one shoulder, matching wider ribbon sash and bow on low waistline. Short cotton socks. Heelless silk shoes with buttoned bar straps and round toes.

Hats 1883–1899

1 8-year-old girl, *c.* 1884. Stiffened felt hat, brim with deep turned-up edge and tall flat-topped crown trimmed with wide contrast-colour petersham ribbon band and large ostrich feather on one side held with brooch and pin. 2 10-year-old girl, *c.* 1896. Silk organza hat with wide pleated double brim under silk satin ribbon band with silk flower trim, pleating repeated above band, spotted silk tulle crown. 3 3-year-old boy, *c.* 1883. Brimless velvet hat, large unstructured crown gathered onto wide band with pin-tucked decoration. 4 6-year-old boy, *c.* 1899. Natural straw hat, wide brim with swept-up edge bound with coloured silk, matching band and bow trim on shallow domed crown. 5 8-year-old boy, *c.* 1887. Natural straw hat, wide turned-down brim, tall domed crown with crease from centre front to centre back, petersham ribbon band with long trailing ends at back. 6 12-year-old boy, *c.* 1899. Natural straw boater, wide flat stiffened brim, matching shallow flat-topped crown with striped ribbon band and bow trim on one side. 7 Baby, *c.* 1895. Fine stiffened cotton voile bonnet with frilled brim, back and skirt edged with gathered lace, coloured silk trimmings and ribbon fastenings. 8 10-year-old boy, *c.* 1898. Wool tweed cap with wide peak and sectioned crown with central self-fabric covered button trim. 9 8-year-old boy, *c.* 1894. Brimless stiffened felt hat, shallow domed crown with central contrast-colour pompon trim, matching colour of silk piping and binding on edges of wide band and long trailing ends at back. 10 12-year-old girl, *c.* 1893. Natural straw hat, wide wavy brim with wired edge, silk flower and leaf decoration, shallow domed crown with silk ribbon band, matching wired loops of ribbon bows. 11 10-year-old girl, *c.* 1883. Silk-covered bonnet, wide brim edged with contrast-colour silk, matching swathed band and loops on side of tall flat-topped feather-trimmed crown, colour of silk repeated in ribbon ties. 12 8-year-old girl, *c.* 1887. Brimless striped silk hat, tall padded crown gathered onto wide stiffened contrast-colour striped silk band, matching padded bow trim on side front. 13 5-year-old boy, *c.* 1886. Stiffened felt hat, wide flat brim with wired edge, tall flat-topped crown with contrast-colour silk band, matching diagonal trimming, large covered button and trailing ends on one side. 14 10-year-old girl, *c.* 1890. Brimless striped silk hat, outsized sectioned padded crown with self-fabric central button trim, gathered onto stiffened band.

Hats 1900–1916

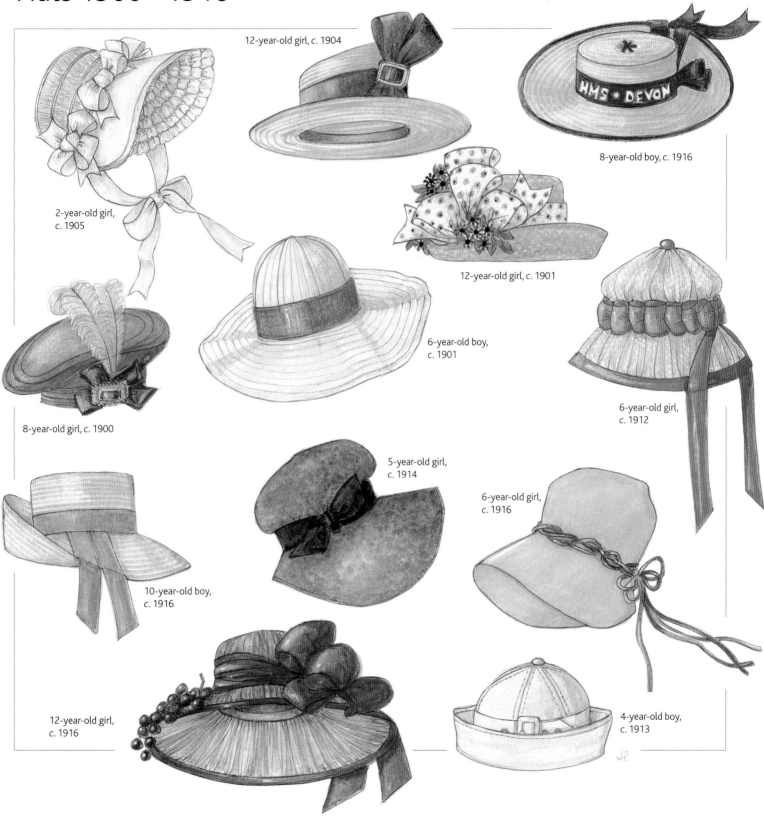

12-year-old girl, c. 1904

8-year-old boy, c. 1916

2-year-old girl, c. 1905

12-year-old girl, c. 1901

6-year-old boy, c. 1901

6-year-old girl, c. 1912

8-year-old girl, c. 1900

5-year-old girl, c. 1914

6-year-old girl, c. 1916

10-year-old boy, c. 1916

12-year-old girl, c. 1916

4-year-old boy, c. 1913

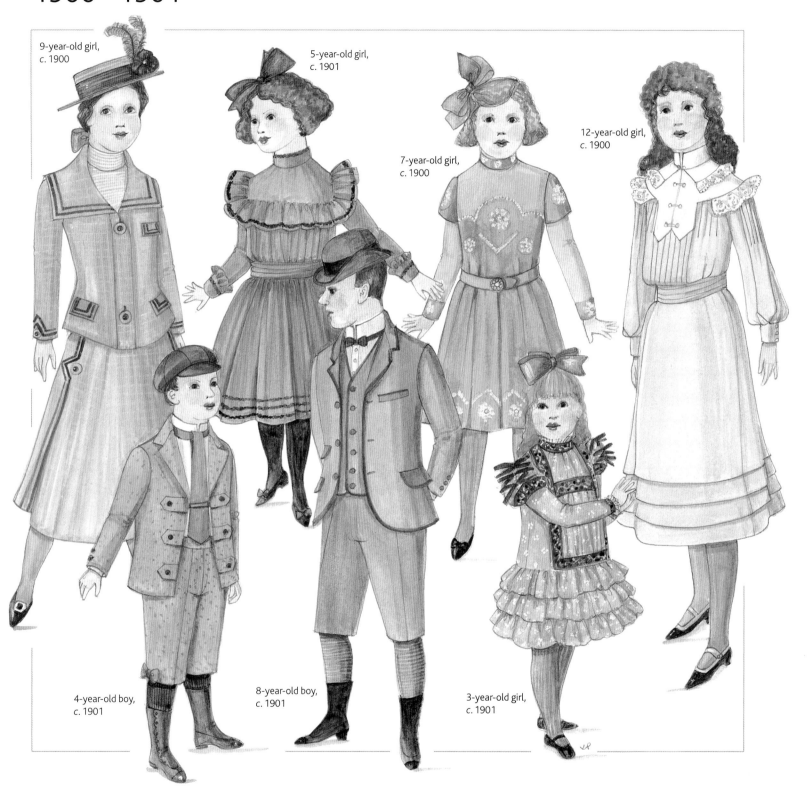

9-year-old girl,
c. 1900

5-year-old girl,
c. 1901

7-year-old girl,
c. 1900

12-year-old girl,
c. 1900

4-year-old boy,
c. 1901

8-year-old boy,
c. 1901

3-year-old girl,
c. 1901

1902 –1903

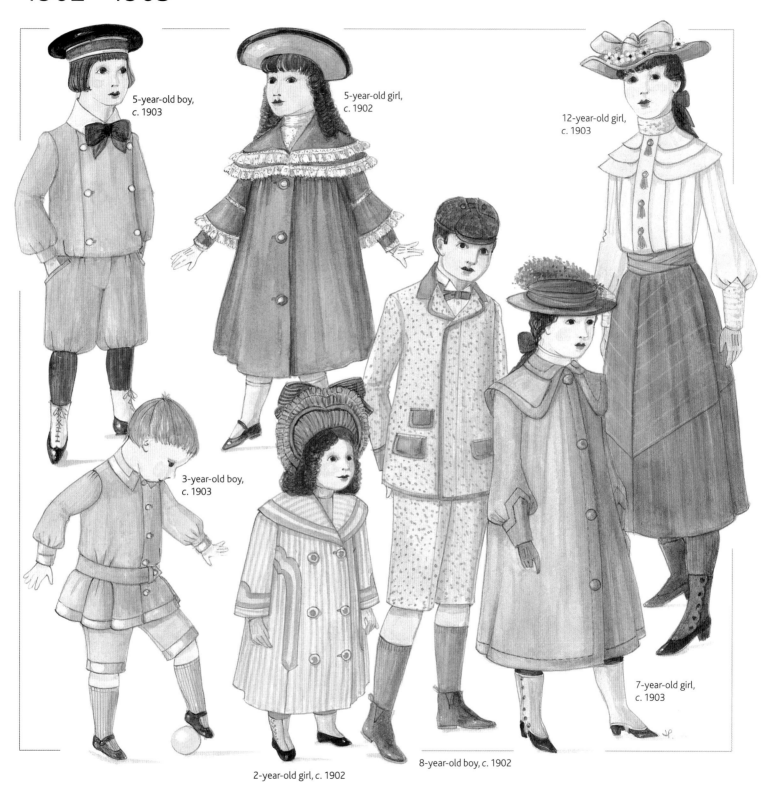

5-year-old boy,
c. 1903

5-year-old girl,
c. 1902

12-year-old girl,
c. 1903

3-year-old boy,
c. 1903

7-year-old girl,
c. 1903

2-year-old girl, c. 1902

8-year-old boy, c. 1902

1904–1905

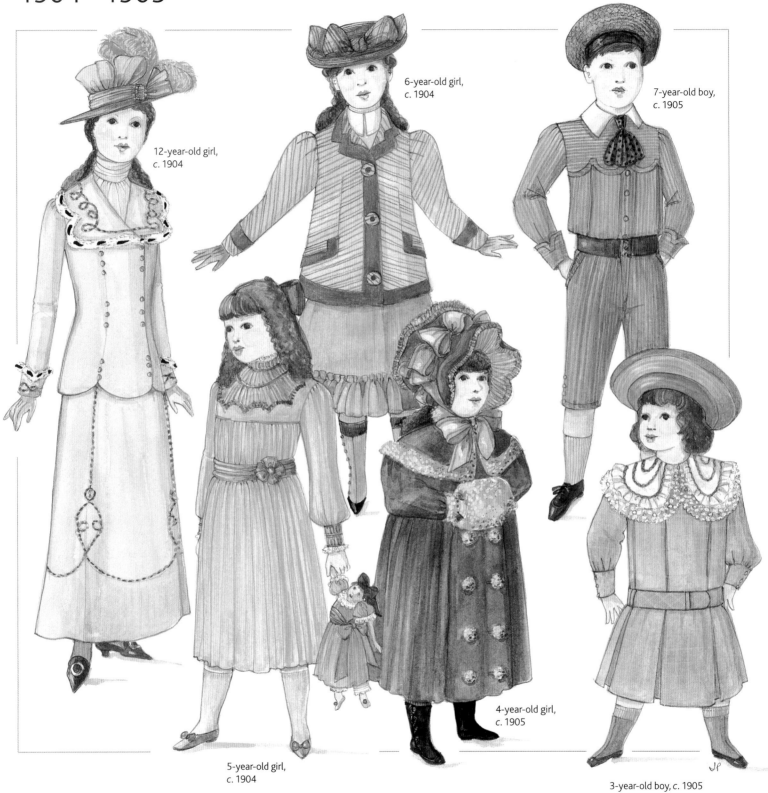

12-year-old girl,
c. 1904

6-year-old girl,
c. 1904

7-year-old boy,
c. 1905

5-year-old girl,
c. 1904

4-year-old girl,
c. 1905

3-year-old boy, *c.* 1905

1906 –1908

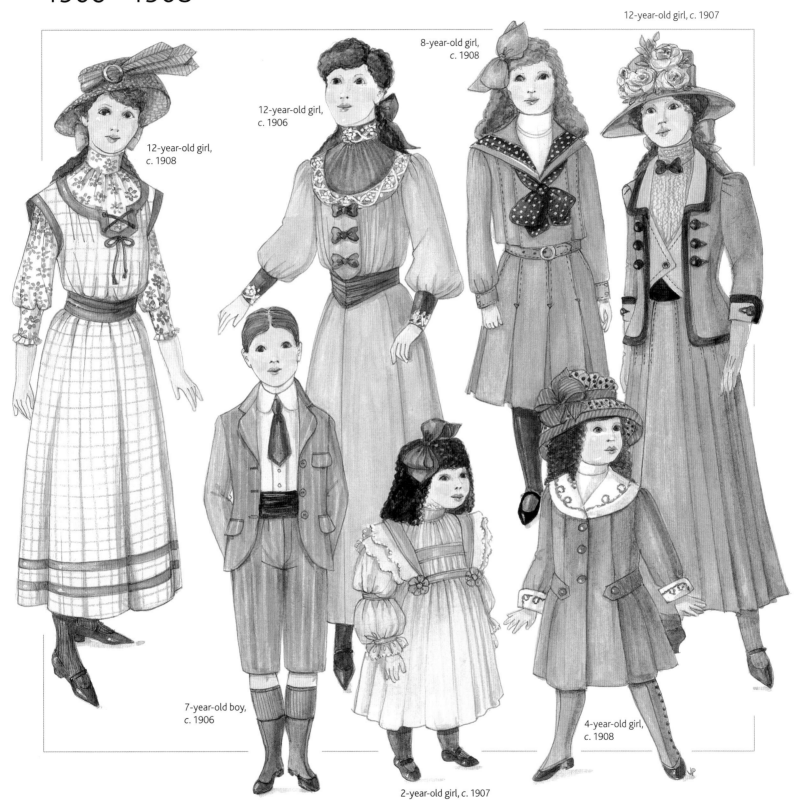

12-year-old girl, c. 1907

8-year-old girl, c. 1908

12-year-old girl, c. 1906

12-year-old girl, c. 1908

7-year-old boy, c. 1906

2-year-old girl, c. 1907

4-year-old girl, c. 1908

1909–1910

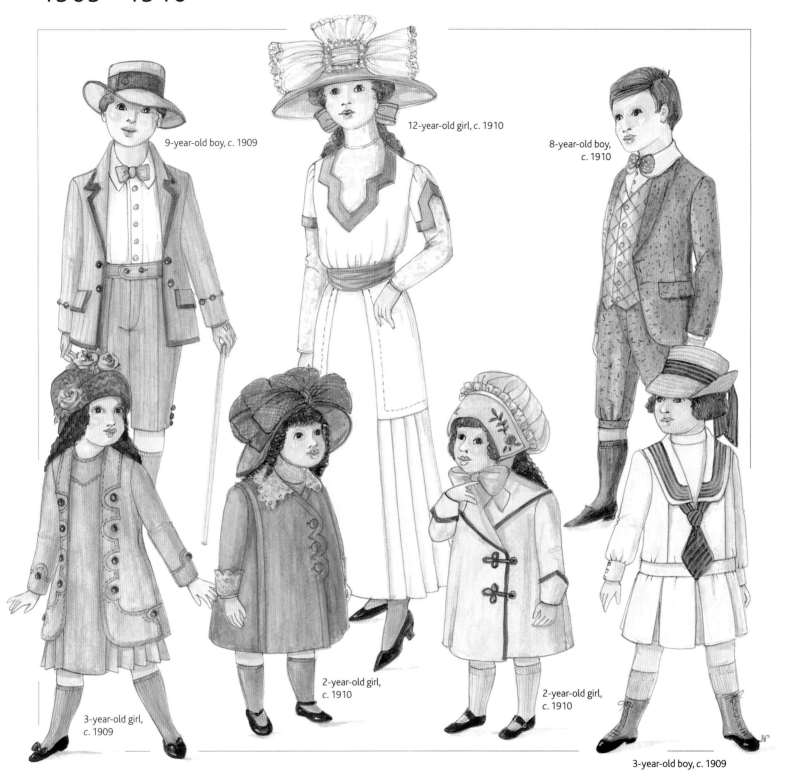

9-year-old boy, c. 1909

12-year-old girl, c. 1910

8-year-old boy, c. 1910

3-year-old girl, c. 1909

2-year-old girl, c. 1910

2-year-old girl, c. 1910

3-year-old boy, c. 1909

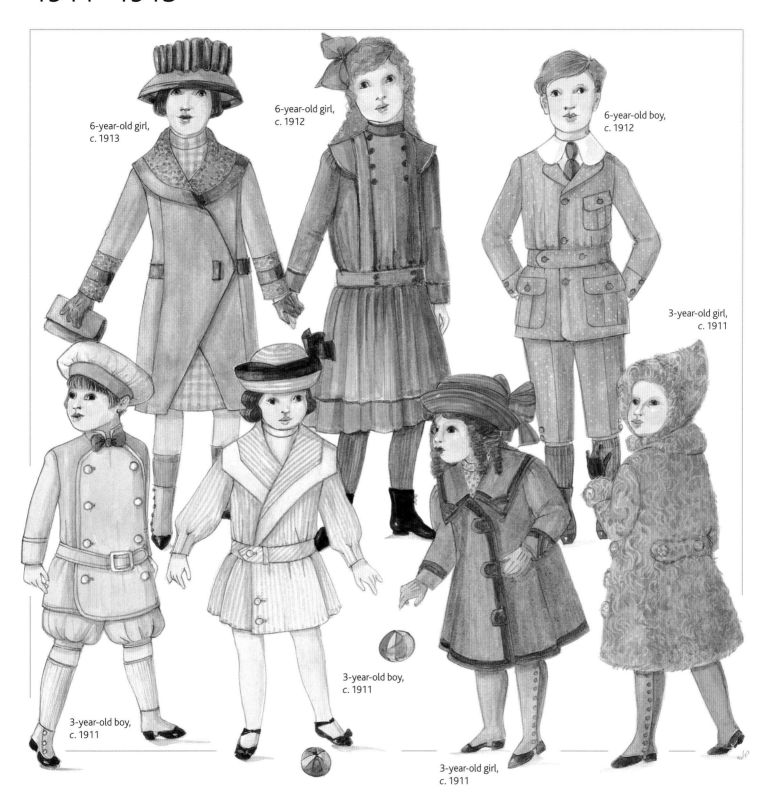

6-year-old girl,
c. 1913

6-year-old girl,
c. 1912

6-year-old boy,
c. 1912

3-year-old girl,
c. 1911

3-year-old boy,
c. 1911

3-year-old boy,
c. 1911

3-year-old girl,
c. 1911

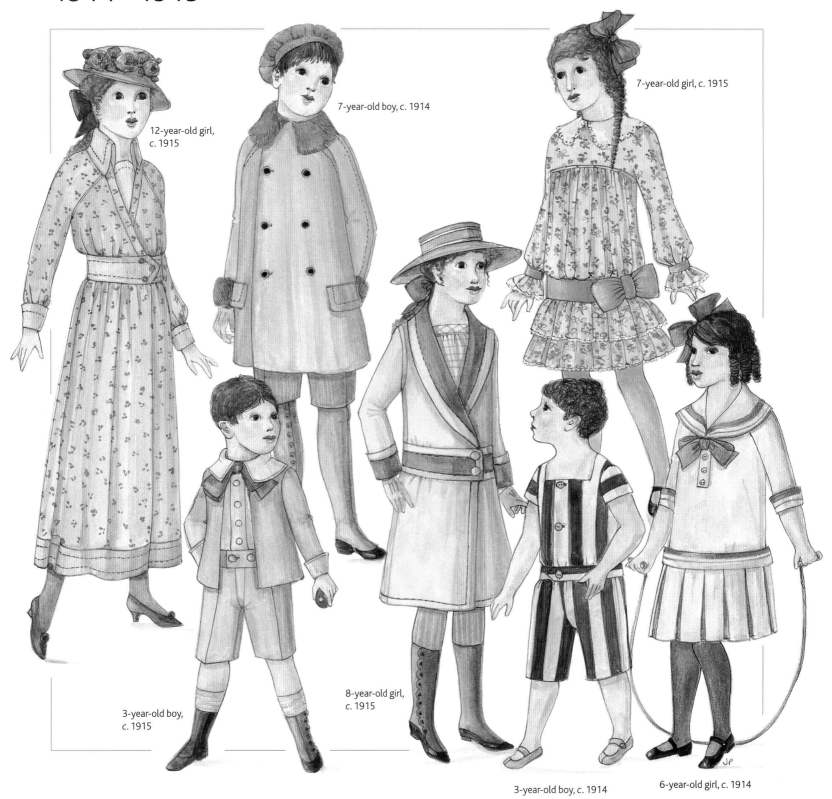

12-year-old girl, c. 1915

7-year-old boy, c. 1914

7-year-old girl, c. 1915

3-year-old boy, c. 1915

8-year-old girl, c. 1915

3-year-old boy, c. 1914

6-year-old girl, c. 1914

1916–1918

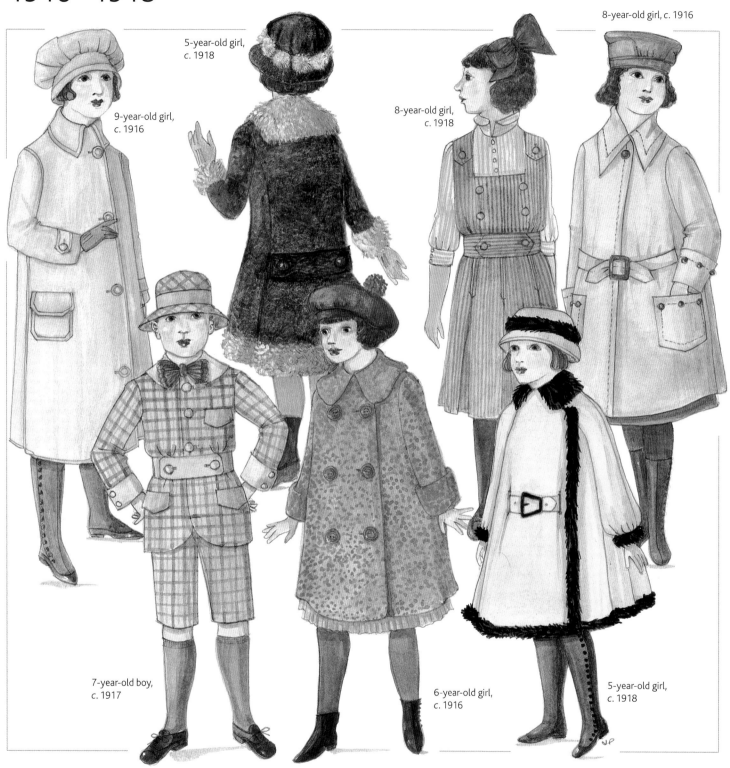

9-year-old girl,
c. 1916

5-year-old girl,
c. 1918

8-year-old girl, c. 1916

8-year-old girl,
c. 1918

7-year-old boy,
c. 1917

6-year-old girl,
c. 1916

5-year-old girl,
c. 1918

1919 –1920

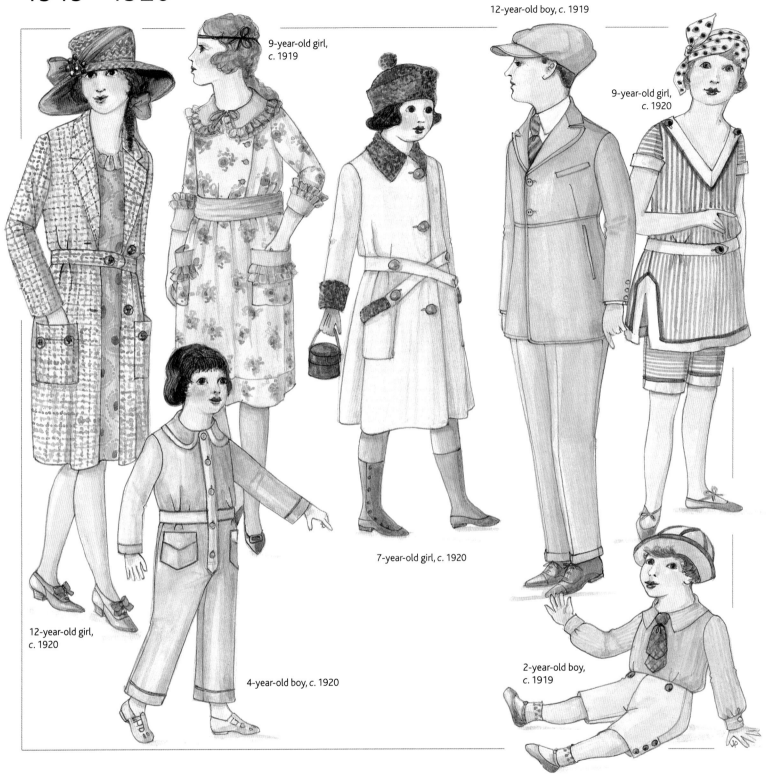

9-year-old girl, c. 1919

12-year-old boy, c. 1919

9-year-old girl, c. 1920

7-year-old girl, c. 1920

12-year-old girl, c. 1920

4-year-old boy, c. 1920

2-year-old boy, c. 1919

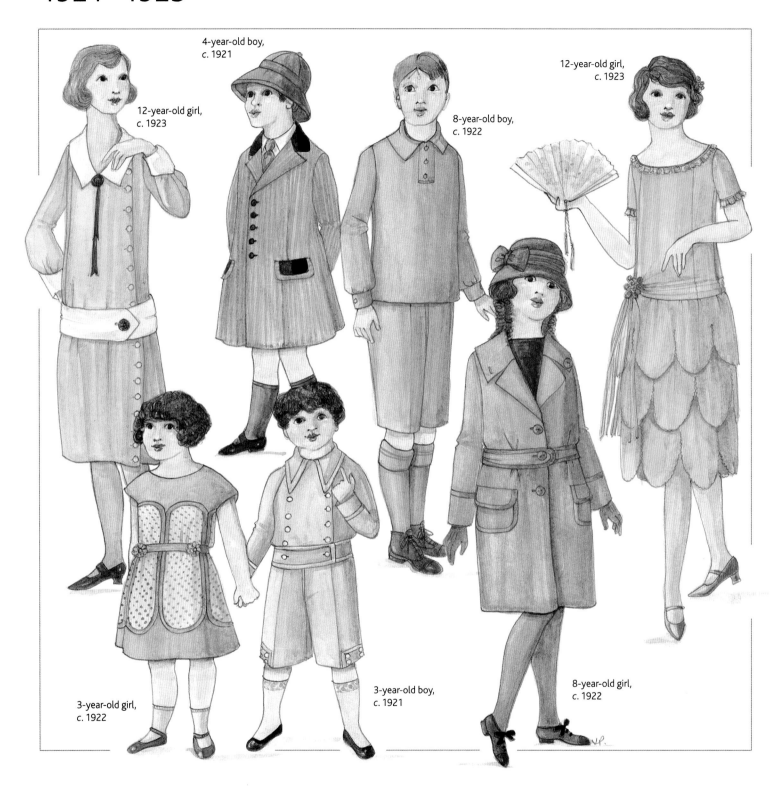

4-year-old boy,
c. 1921

12-year-old girl,
c. 1923

12-year-old girl,
c. 1923

8-year-old boy,
c. 1922

3-year-old girl,
c. 1922

3-year-old boy,
c. 1921

8-year-old girl,
c. 1922

1924–1925

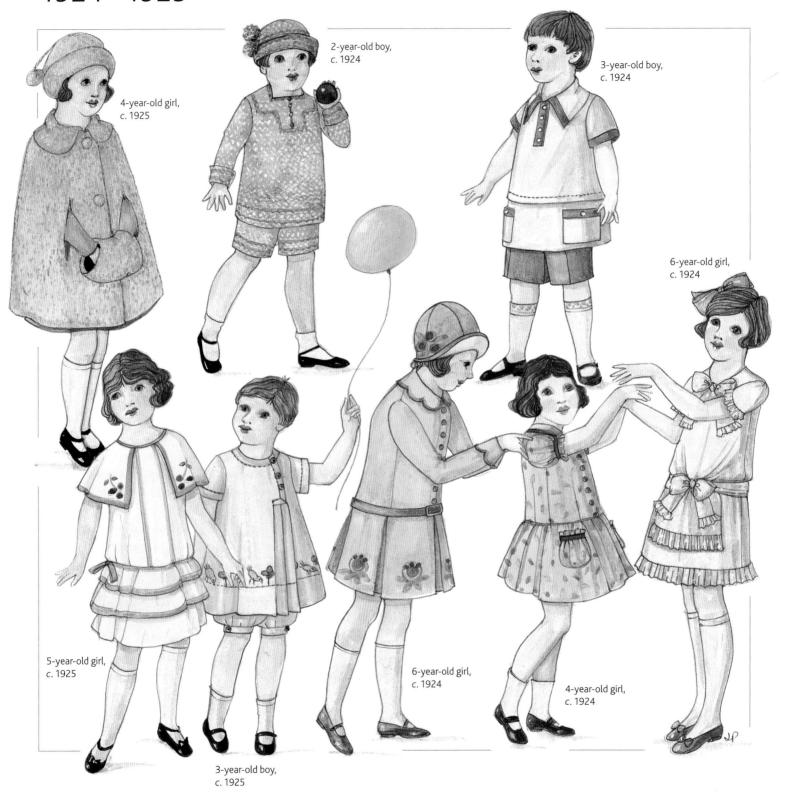

4-year-old girl,
c. 1925

2-year-old boy,
c. 1924

3-year-old boy,
c. 1924

6-year-old girl,
c. 1924

5-year-old girl,
c. 1925

3-year-old boy,
c. 1925

6-year-old girl,
c. 1924

4-year-old girl,
c. 1924

1926–1928

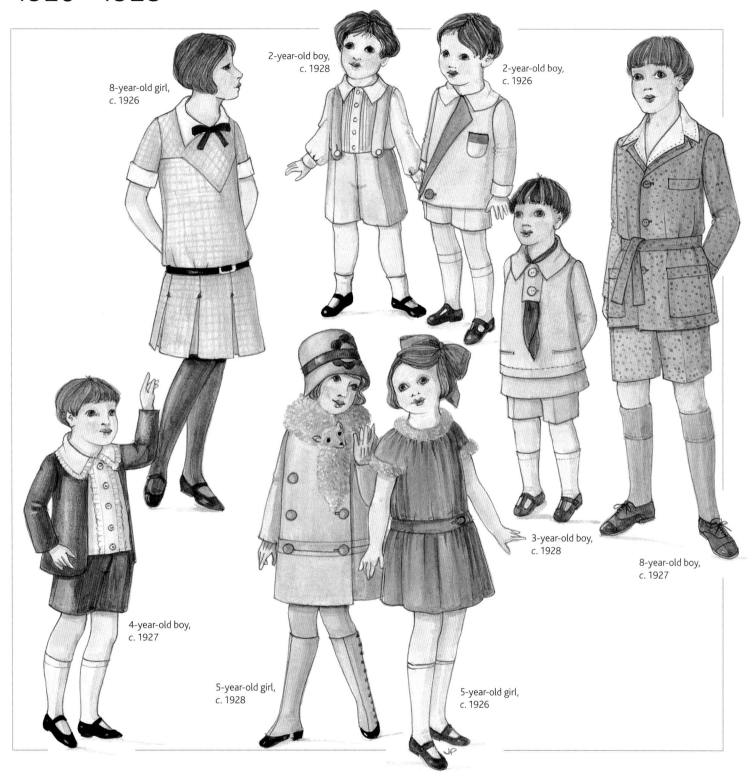

8-year-old girl,
c. 1926

2-year-old boy,
c. 1928

2-year-old boy,
c. 1926

4-year-old boy,
c. 1927

5-year-old girl,
c. 1928

5-year-old girl,
c. 1926

3-year-old boy,
c. 1928

8-year-old boy,
c. 1927

1929 – 1930

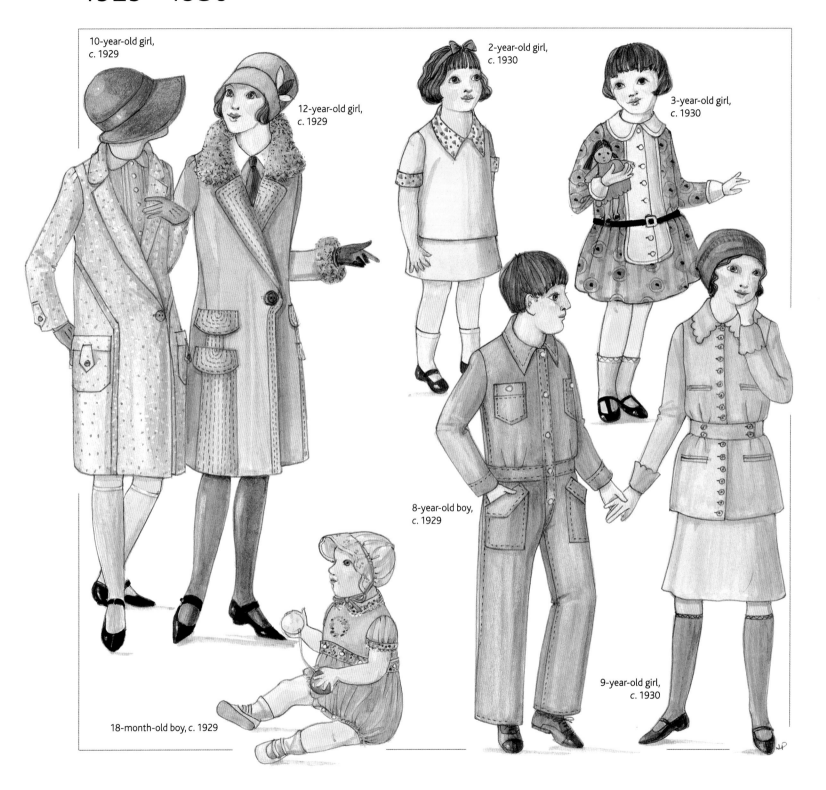

10-year-old girl,
c. 1929

12-year-old girl,
c. 1929

2-year-old girl,
c. 1930

3-year-old girl,
c. 1930

8-year-old boy,
c. 1929

18-month-old boy, c. 1929

9-year-old girl,
c. 1930

1931–1933

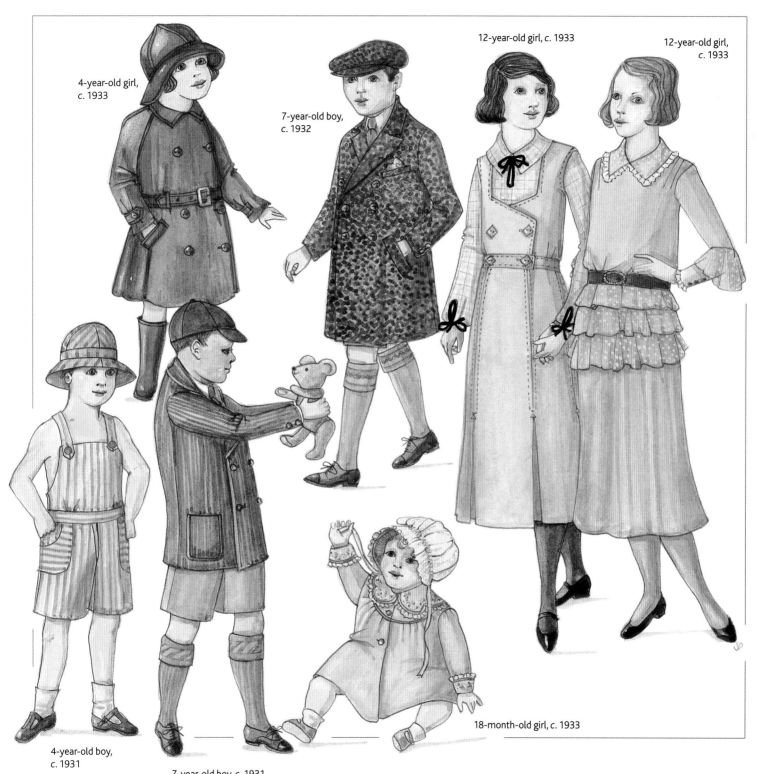

4-year-old girl,
c. 1933

7-year-old boy,
c. 1932

12-year-old girl, c. 1933

12-year-old girl,
c. 1933

4-year-old boy,
c. 1931

7-year-old boy, c. 1931

18-month-old girl, c. 1933

Hats 1917–1933

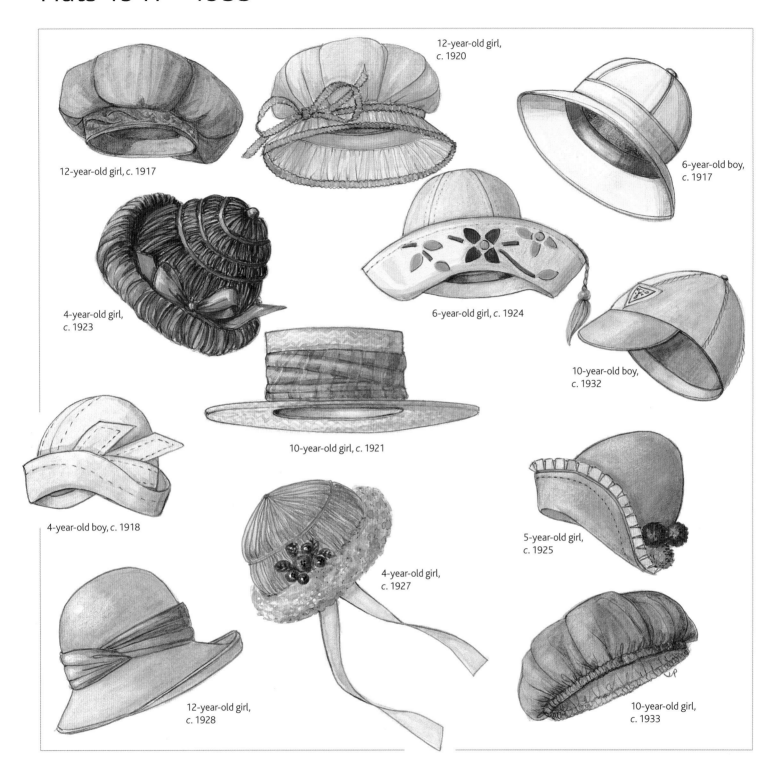

12-year-old girl, c. 1917

12-year-old girl,
c. 1920

6-year-old boy,
c. 1917

4-year-old girl,
c. 1923

6-year-old girl, c. 1924

10-year-old boy,
c. 1932

10-year-old girl, c. 1921

4-year-old boy, c. 1918

5-year-old girl,
c. 1925

12-year-old girl,
c. 1928

4-year-old girl,
c. 1927

10-year-old girl,
c. 1933

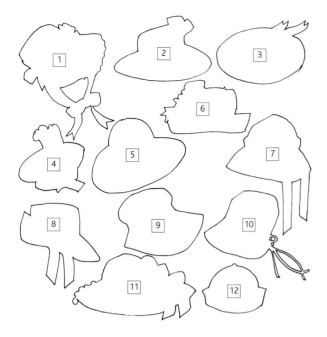

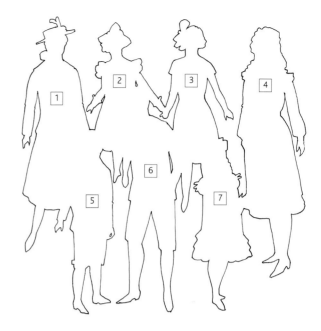

Hats 1900 –1916

1 2-year-old girl, *c.* 1905. Silk-covered bonnet, deep front brim lined with rows of contrast-colour frilled silk, colour repeated in piping between bands of ruching on tall crown, loops and ribbon bows circling crown and ribbon ties under chin. 2 12-year-old girl, *c.* 1904. Natural straw hat, wide flat brim with wired edge, tall asymmetric crown with wide ribbon band, matching looped side trim pulled through cut steel buckle. 3 8-year-old boy, *c.* 1916. Stiffened natural straw hat, wide brim, edge bound with ribbon, matching lettered band around shallow flat-topped crown, motif on top crown, loops and trailing ends. 4 8-year-old girl, *c.* 1900. Brimless wool hat, wide band with top-stitched detail, matching rows of stitching on edges of asymmetric flat crown, two-feather trim on one side from above looped contrast-colour silk ribbon bow and cut steel buckle. 5 6-year-old boy, *c.* 1901. Stiffened cotton hat, wide unstructured brim with rows of top-stitched detail, matching tall sectioned crown, wide contrast-colour leather hatband. 6 12-year-old girl, *c.* 1901. Stiffened natural plaited straw hat, narrow turned-up brim with wired edge, shallow flat-topped crown with wide embroidered ribbon band, matching wired loops among silk flowers on front of hat. 7 6-year-old girl, *c.* 1912. Checked cotton hat, narrow turned-down ruched brim with wired edge, wide contrast-colour cotton velvet binding, matching covered ball button trim on top of shallow gathered crown and looped hatband with bow and trailing ends at back. 8 10-year-old boy, *c.* 1916. Stiffened natural straw hat, wide brim turned down at front and up at back, tall flat-topped crown with wide ribbon band and trailing ends to one side. 9 5-year-old girl, *c.* 1914. Textured wool hat, bonnet-shaped brim, wide at front and narrow at back with wired edge, shallow unstructured crown, wide ribbon band and side knot with pointed ends. 10 6-year-old girl, *c.* 1916. Stiffened felt hat, bonnet-shaped brim, wide at front and narrow at back, tall crown, blocked to shape, hatband in three colours of twisted ribbon with looped bows and trailing ends at back. 11 12-year-old girl, *c.* 1916. Silk-covered hat, wide ruched brim and lining, wired edge with wide contrast-colour silk binding, matching draped hatband and looped decoration on one side with trailing ends, tall domed crown, wax fruit balancing trim. 12 4-year-old boy, *c.* 1913. Stiffened cotton hat, narrow brim turned up all around top-stitched edge, matching shallow sectioned crown with self-fabric button trim on top, wide contrast-colour leather hatband with buckle and eyelet hole trim.

1900 –1901

1 9-year-old girl, *c.* 1900. Checked wool suit: unfitted hip-length jacket, single-breasted strap fastening with decorative button under shoulder-wide sailor collar and one above hemline, matching detail on hems of long sleeves and on side panel seams at hip level in flared mid-calf-length skirt, single breast flap pocket and matching flap pockets above hemline of jacket, trimmed with contrast-colour wool braid, repeated on collar, sleeve hems and side panel seams in skirt. Silk blouse with stand collar. Stiffened straw boater, flat-topped crown with ribbon band, matching rosette on one side trimmed with two feathers. Silk stockings. Leather shoes with buckle trim and pointed toes. 2 5-year-old girl, *c.* 1901. Cotton dress, bloused bodice with stand collar, frill-trimmed shoulder-wide yoke, matching edges of cuffs on long sleeves, wide self-fabric waist-sash, knee-length gathered skirt trimmed above hemline with rows of contrast-colour cotton lace braid, repeated on collar, cuffs and edge of yoke frill. Large ribbon bow worn in hair. Cotton stockings. Leather shoes with bow trim above pointed toes and low heels. 3 7-year-old girl, *c.* 1900. Silk party dress with contrast-colour shaped yoke and long fitted undersleeves, stand collar trimmed with lace motifs, matching short oversleeves, sleeve cuffs, fitted bodice and hemline of knee-length skirt, narrow self-fabric waist-belt with clasp fastening. Large ribbon bow worn in hair. Cotton stockings. Leather shoes with bow trim above pointed toes. 4 12-year-old girl, *c.* 1900. Cotton dress, bloused bodice with tucked front panel, contrast-colour stand collar, matching lace-edged sham collar, wide yoke with lace trimming over shoulders and buttoned double-strap front fastening to chest level, long sleeves, with tucked inset panel, gathered into buttoned cuffs, self-fabric tucked waist-sash, knee-length flared panelled skirt with tucks above hemline. Silk stockings. Leather shoes with contrast-colour buttoned bar straps and trimmed edges, pointed toes and low heels. 5 4-year-old boy, *c.* 1901. Two-piece wool tweed suit: edge-to-edge hip-length jacket with buttoned-down sham straps, single strap fastening at low chest level on inside, narrow collar and revers, long sleeves with button trim; knee-length trousers with fly fronts, central creases and bow trim on side seams above hemline. Cotton shirt with stiffened stand collar and long sleeves, worn with long silk necktie. Wool peaked cap with sectioned crown. Ribbed wool stockings. Leather boots with side-button fastenings, pointed toecaps and stacked heels. 6 8-year-old boy, *c.* 1901. Two-piece wool suit: hip-length single-breasted jacket with narrow braid-trimmed collar and revers, matching edges of two flap pockets, small ticket pocket, breast pocket and collarless single-breasted waistcoat, long sleeves with button trim; knee-length trousers with fly fronts and central creases. Cotton shirt with stiffened stand collar, worn with silk bow tie. Stiffened felt bowler hat with curled braid-trimmed brim and tall crown with petersham band. Ribbed wool stockings. Leather boots with side-button fastenings, pointed toecaps and high heels. 7 3-year-old girl, *c.* 1901. Patterned silk party dress, hip-length bodice with ruched central panel edged with embroidered braid, matching stand collar with frilled edge, cuffs with frilled edges on long undersleeves and edges of short puffed and ribbon-trimmed oversleeves, knee-length tiered and gathered skirt. Large ribbon bow worn in hair. Ribbed silk stockings. Heelless satin shoes with buttoned bar straps, leather soles and round toes.

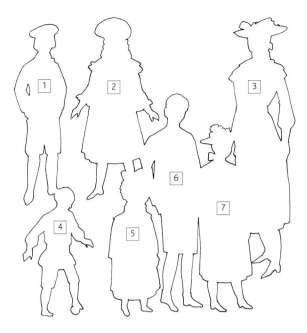

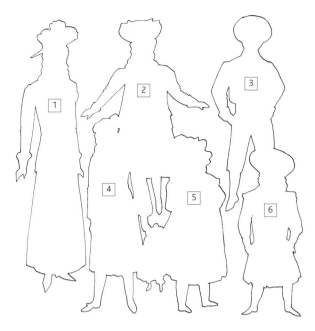

1902 – 1903

1 5-year-old boy, *c.* 1903. Two-piece wool flannel suit: double-breasted bloused jacket, fastening with large pearl buttons, full-length sleeves gathered into cuffs, detachable stiff cotton collar worn with large silk bow tie; breeches gathered at knee level with fly fronts and hip-level pockets. Brimless wool hat, flat beret crown attached to deep contrast-colour band with petersham ribbon trim. Ribbed wool stockings. Ankle-length two-tone leather boots with hooked and laced front fastenings, pointed toes and stacked heels. 2 5-year-old girl, *c.* 1902. Unfitted wool flannel coat, single-breasted fastening with outsized buttons under double shoulder-wide collars edged with gathered lace, matching hems of flared elbow-length oversleeves, wrist-length undersleeves trimmed with border lace. Straw hat, wide turned-up brim edged with braid. Short cotton gloves. Calf-length knitted cotton socks. Leather bar strap shoes with pointed toes and low heels. 3 12-year-old girl, *c.* 1903. Fine cotton blouse, tucked bodice with sham front strap fastening, decorated with tasselled buttons, three-tier shoulder-wide sham collar under lace stand collar, matching deep cuffs on full sleeves. Mid-calf-length striped wool flared skirt with pointed bias-cut panels, front and back, skirt worn with draped silk cummerbund. Dyed fine straw hat with wide wavy brim, bound with contrast-colour silk, matching looped bow on crown, silk flower trim. Short cotton gloves. Long wool stockings. Above-ankle-length leather boots with side-button fastenings, pointed toes and high stacked heels. 4 3-year-old boy, *c.* 1903. Two-piece knitted wool suit: single-breasted hip-length jacket, fastening with pearl buttons under large collar bound in contrast colour, matching cuffs on long sleeves, hems of jacket and knee-length trousers, wide self-fabric belt with pearl button fastening. Knee-length ribbed cotton socks. Heelless leather bar strap shoes with blunt toes. 5 2-year-old girl, *c.* 1902. Long unfitted double-breasted striped wool coat, button fastening under shoulder-wide collar with braid-trimmed edge, matching hems of long flared sleeves and side panel seams. Large hat with turned-up heart-shaped brim trimmed with ruched silk, velvet ribbon and frilled edge, outsized striped silk bow at back. Short cotton gloves. Cotton socks. Above-ankle-length two-tone boots: cloth uppers with side-button fastenings and contrast-colour heelless leather shoes with blunt toes. 6 8-year-old boy, *c.* 1902. Two-piece wool tweed suit: hip-length jacket with concealed single-breasted fastening under fly fastening, contrast-colour velvet collar, matching flap pockets and cuffs on long sleeves, braid edges and detail; knee-length trousers with central crease. Wool tweed peaked cap with ear flaps buttoned onto top of crown. Cotton shirt, stiff wing collar worn with silk bow tie. Knee-length wool socks. Ankle-length elastic-sided leather boots with back pull tapes, round toes and low heels. 7 7-year-old girl, *c.* 1903. Unfitted knee-length wool coat, single-breasted fastening with outsized buttons from under collar and shoulder-wide cape, long sleeves gathered into pointed stitched cuffs, top-stitched hems, edges and detail. Cloth hat with wired brim, low flat-topped crown with draped band, matching colour of ostrich feather trim. Short cloth gloves. Wool stockings. Cloth spats with side-button fastenings and stirrups under feet of leather shoes with pointed toes and high heels.

1904 – 1905

1 12-year-old girl, *c.* 1904. Fine wool two-piece suit: hip-length double-breasted jacket, fastening with small self-fabric covered buttons in sets of three, shoulder-wide collar trimmed with ermine, matching edges of shaped cuffs on full-length sleeves; ankle-length flared skirt decorated with fancy braid, repeated on collar and cuffs. Silk blouse with high collar. Dyed straw hat with wide brim, tall crown covered with draped silk band threaded through a cut metal buckle, trimmed with matching loops of silk and three curled ostrich feathers. Short leather gloves. Ribbel wool stockings. Leather shoes, high tongues trimmed with silver buckles, pointed toes and shaped high heels. 2 6-year-old girl, *c.* 1904. Hip-length striped wool jacket with unfitted bodice, single-breasted fastening with outsized self-fabric covered buttons from high collar and revers, hip-level flap pockets, leg-of-mutton sleeves with deep cuffs, edges and detail bound with velvet. Knee-length wool skirt with frilled hemline. Cotton blouse with high stiff shirt-style collar. Straw hat with wide brim turned up on edge, shallow crown with striped silk ribbon bow trim. Short leather gloves. Knee-length knitted wool stockings above cloth spats with side-button fastenings, leather shoes with pointed toes. 3 7-year-old boy, *c.* 1905. Striped cotton shirt with centre-front buttoned strap fastening, scalloped yoke seam, matching cuffs on full-length sleeves. Knee-length trousers in matching fabric with hip-level pockets, front fly fastening and button detail on outside leg seams above hemlines, trousers worn with wide leather belt with clasp fastening. Shirt worn with stiff collar in contrast colour and spotted silk necktie. Hat with turned-up straw brim set onto wide stiffened petersham ribbon band. Short knitted cotton stockings. Lace-up leather shoes with square toes and stacked heels. 4 5-year-old girl, *c.* 1904. Knee-length silk dress with bloused bodice from under yoke seam, scalloped neckline edged with contrast-colour ruching and filled with gathered bands of second contrast colour and piped with first, matching waist-sash with rosette trim, lace-edged stand collar and cuffs on full-length gathered sleeves, full skirt. Ribbon bow with trailing ends worn in hair at back. Knee-length knitted cotton stockings. Leather shoes with low heels and bow trim above pointed toes. 5 4-year-old girl, *c.* 1905. Below-knee-length velvet coat, double-breasted fastening with outsized fur-covered buttons, matching edge of attached shoulder cape, collar, cuffs of long sleeves and hand muff. Silk bonnet with outsized wired brim and outsized crown, lined and trimmed with contrast-colour pleated and ruched silk, wide striped silk ribbon loops and bows, matching ties under chin. Long leather boots with side-button fastenings, pointed toes and low heels. 6 3-year-old boy, *c.* 1905. Checked silk frock with hip-length box-pleated bodice, matching attached knee-length skirt with wide belt, full-length sleeves with buttoned cuffs, shoulder-wide plain cotton collar with three rows of braid trim, frilled edge and wide lace trim. Three-colour straw hat with wide turned-up brim. Short knitted cotton stockings above cloth spats, leather shoes with square toes and low heels.

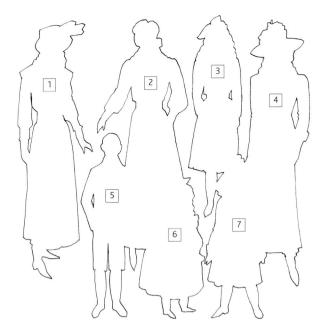

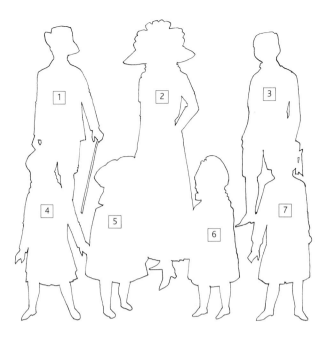

1906 – 1908

1 12-year-old girl, *c.* 1908. Checked cotton sleeveless pinafore dress with bloused bodice, low scooped neckline with laced detail on centre front, edges bound with plain colour cotton satin, matching armholes, deep waist-sash and two inset bands above hem of ankle-length gathered skirt. Patterned cotton blouse with high stand collar and three-quarter-length sleeves gathered into deep cuffs with pleated hems. Large straw hat with asymmetric brim and high crown, wide band and sham feathers in matching fabric pulled through large buckle. Cotton stockings. Leather bar strap shoes with pointed toes and stacked heels. 2 12-year-old girl, *c.* 1906. Fine wool dress, bloused bodice decorated with three contrast-colour silk bows on centre front, matching fabric of blouse in-fill with stand collar, deep cuffs on long sleeves and pleated waistband, ankle-length flared skirt, dress collar and cuffs and blouse collar decorated with fancy braid. Hair tied back with large ribbon bow. Cotton stockings. Leather bar strap shoes with pointed toes. 3 8-year-old girl, *c.* 1908. Cotton dress, bloused bodice with sewn pleats continued into knee-length skirt, long sleeves with buttoned cuffs, self-fabric belt with metal buckle, large sailor-style collar trimmed with contrast-colour spotted cotton, matching scarf tied into large bow at front under collar. Plain blouse with stand collar. Large ribbon bow worn in hair on one side. Cotton stockings. Leather bar strap shoes with pointed toes. 4 12-year-old girl, *c.* 1907. Three-piece fine wool suit: fitted jacket cut to be worn open, contrast-colour collar, matching cuffs of three-quarter-length sleeves and waistcoat with single button fastening, jacket edges and detail bound in second contrast colour, colour repeated in buttons, button holes and waist-sash; ankle-length skirt with knife pleats on either side, sewn down to hip level. Patterned silk blouse with contrast-colour silk bow tie worn under high stand collar. Straw hat, wide brim and tall crown with deep ribbon band, trimmed with large silk roses. Ribbon bow worn in hair at back. Long kid gloves. Knitted stockings. Leather bar strap shoes with pointed toes and shaped heels. 5 7-year-old boy, *c.* 1906. Two-piece striped fine wool flannel suit: single-breasted jacket with three button fastening, narrow collar and revers, long sleeves and three flap pockets; knee-length trousers with fly fronts, wide contrast-colour silk waist-sash. Cotton shirt with buttoned strap fastening, stiff collar worn with short necktie. Knee-length wool socks. Cloth spats, leather shoes with round toes and stacked heels. 6 2-year-old girl, *c.* 1907. Silk dress with high waist bodice gathered from under high stand collar, velvet epaulettes, matching horizontal straps across chest and high waist trimmed with rosettes continued in bands at elbow and wrist level above frilled cuffs, two bias-cut frills under epaulettes trimmed with narrow lace, lace edging repeated on cuffs and collar, gathered knee-length skirt. Silk ribbon bow worn in hair on one side. Cotton stockings. Heelless leather bar strap shoes with round toes. 7 4-year-old girl, *c.* 1908. Single-breasted velvet coat with three button fastening, decorative hip-level belt buttoned on side fronts above pleated skirts, shoulder-wide contrast-colour silk collar trimmed with fancy braid, matching cuffs on long sleeves. Silk blouse with stand collar. Large hat with wide turned-down brim covered with spotted tulle and bound in striped silk, matching gathered crown, band and bow trim on one side. Knee-length cloth spats with side-button fastenings, leather shoes with round toes and stacked heels.

1909 – 1910

1 9-year-old boy, *c.* 1909. Two-piece striped cotton suit: long jacket cut to be worn open, with two button trim on either side, collar and revers bound with plain cotton, matching flap pockets, long sleeves, sewn cuffs trimmed with buttons, matching detail on side seams above hems of knee-length trousers, wide waistband with button fastenings above fly fronts. Plain cotton shirt with buttoned strap fastening and stiff collar, worn with silk bow tie. Straw hat, wide brim turned up on one side and tall flat-topped crown, wide petersham band with button trim. Short kid gloves. Walking stick. Knee-length wool socks. 2 12-year-old girl, *c.* 1910. Ankle-length linen dress with bloused bodice, low shaped neckline with wide contrast-colour binding, matching hems and cut-out detail on short sleeves and wide waist-sash, flared skirt with plain front panel, top-stitched side panels to low hip level, above knife pleats. Lace blouse with high stand collar and long sleeves. Large straw hat, wide brim with bound edge, crown decorated with outsized lace-trimmed bow, threaded through large metal buckle set with stones. Large ribbon bow worn in hair at back. Flesh-coloured silk stockings. Leather shoes with low-cut fronts, pointed toes and shaped heels. 3 8-year-old boy, *c.* 1910. Two-piece wool tweed suit: single-breasted jacket with narrow shawl collar, long sleeves with two-button trim above hems and flap pockets; breeches gathered into wide bands on knee level, fly fronts. Single-breasted collarless checked wool waistcoat. Cotton shirt, stiff collar worn with silk bow tie. Knee-length wool socks. Leather shoes with high tongues, square toes and stacked heels. 4 3-year-old girl, *c.* 1909. Collarless silk dress with unfitted bodice, cut without waist seam, high V-shaped yoke-seam top-stitched detail, knee-length skirt with knife-pleated side panels. Short edge-to-edge coat in matching fabric, trimmed with large buttons and fancy top-stitched seams, repeated on cuffs of long sleeves. Straw hat with turned-back brim and tall crown trimmed with silk flowers and leaves. Knee-length cotton socks. Heelless leather shoes trimmed with bows above pointed toes. 5 2-year-old girl, *c.* 1910. Unfitted knee-length velvet coat, single-breasted fastening with three large buttons between scallops on front edge, raised panel seams on each from shoulder to hem, long sleeves with lace cuffs, matching collar, dress with high stand collar. Straw hat, wide brim edged with satin, matching outsized bows covering crown. Knee-length cotton socks. Heelless leather shoes with front buttoned bar straps and round toes. 6 2-year-old girl, *c.* 1910. Unfitted knee-length linen coat, double-breasted wrap-over front, fastening with fancy braid and two buttons, matching front edges, cuffs on long sleeves and edges of shoulder-wide collar. Silk bonnet with gathered crown and embroidered turned-back brim with contrast-colour frilled edge, matching bindings and bow tie under chin. Knee-length cotton socks. Heelless leather shoes with side-button bar straps and round toes. 7 3-year-old boy, *c.* 1909. Linen dress with unfitted bodice above hip-level inset belt, long sleeves with buttoned cuffs, long collar trimmed with contrast colour, matching necktie, knee-length box-pleated skirt, undershirt with stand collar in matching fabric. Straw hat, wide brim turned up at back, tall flat-topped crown with wide band and trailing ends at back. Knee-length cotton socks. Lace-up boots with cloth tops, leather shoes, round toes and stacked heels.

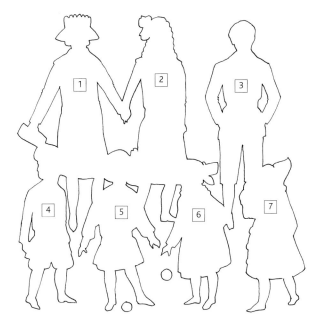
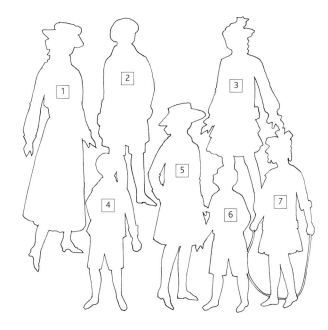

1911–1913

1 6-year-old girl, *c.* 1913. Knee-length fine wool coat, cut-away wrap-over front with concealed fastening at low waist level, shoulder-wide astrakhan collar with contrast-colour velvet binding, matching deep cuffs on long sleeves, velvet repeated on sham belt, threaded from back though side panel seams to front. Knee-length checked wool dress with stand collar. Straw hat with turned-down brim, edge bound with contrast-colour velvet, matching pleated band covering crown. Short leather gloves, matching purse. Knitted cotton socks. Ankle-length cloth spats with side-button fastening, leather shoes with pointed toes.

2 6-year-old girl, *c.* 1912. Cotton satin dress, stand collar with contrast-colour bound edge, matching epaulettes, cuffs on long sleeves, wide tucks on either side front of bloused bodice, covered buttons on upper bodice and hip-level belt and inset piping above hemline of gathered knee-length skirt. Large ribbon bow worn in hair on one side. Long knitted cotton stockings. Ankle-length leather boots with laced fastenings and low stacked heels. 3 6-year-old boy, *c.* 1912. Two-piece flecked wool suit: single-breasted jacket with rounded revers, buttoned waist-belt, long sleeves, sewn cuffs with button detail, three patch pockets with box pleats and buttoned-down flaps; knee-length trousers with central creases and button detail on outside seams above hems. Cotton shirt with large stiffened collar worn over jacket, silk necktie with large knot. Long knitted wool stockings. Leather ankle boots with laced fastenings and square toes. 4 3-year-old boy, *c.* 1911. Two-piece cotton suit: long double-breasted jacket, fastening with pearl buttons, matching buckle on hip-belt, stand collar worn with bow tie, long sleeves with top-stitched cuffs, matching other edges, hems and detail; breeches gathered into wide bands at knee level. Brimless cotton hat with large crown gathered onto wide contrast-colour band. Knee-length knitted cotton socks. Short cloth spats with side-button fastenings, leather shoes with round toes and stacked heels. 5 3-year-old boy, *c.* 1911. Striped cotton coat with concealed single-breasted fastening, plus two decorative buttons above hemline of full skirts, long shoulder-wide collar with deep contrast-colour binding, matching shirt with stand collar, low belt threaded through loop on centre front and buttoned on one side, long sleeves with vertical tucks at wrist level to form cuffs. Straw hat, turned-back brim with wide contrast-colour binding, matching band and rosette on edge of large crown. Long cotton stockings. Heelless leather bar strap shoes with button fastening on front, bow trim above round toes. 6 3-year-old girl, *c.* 1911. Unfitted knee-length wool coat, single-breasted fastening with three large buttons, shoulder-wide collar with contrast-colour braid trim, matching cuffs on long sleeves, hems and edges. Coat worn over spotted cotton dress with stand collar. Felt hat, wide turned-back brim bound with contrast-colour silk, matching band and detail on back of large crown. Short leather gloves. Knee-length cloth spats with side-button fastenings, leather shoes with pointed toes and stacked heels. 7 3-year-old girl, *c.* 1911. Unfitted knee-length fur coat with large collar, single-breasted fastening with fur-covered buttons, matching buttons on half-belt at back and cuffs on long sleeves. Fur bonnet with deep roll brim, pointed crown and ties under chin. Short leather gloves. Knee-length cloth spats with side-button fastenings, leather shoes with round toes and stacked heels.

1914–1915

1 12-year-old girl, *c.* 1915. Mid-calf-length printed cotton dress with wrap-over bodice, self-bound edges forming low neckline with contrast-colour in-fill, matching high collar, cuffs on long raglan sleeves, bound hem of full skirt and wide belt with three button fastening, top-stitched detail. Straw hat with wide brim and large low crown trimmed with silk flowers and ribbon bows. Large ribbon bow worn in hair at back. Knitted silk stockings. Leather shoes with high heels and rosette trim above pointed toes. 2 7-year-old boy, *c.* 1914. Short double-breasted wool topcoat with large flap pockets, deep fur collar, matching cuffs on long raglan sleeves. Knee-length striped wool trousers. Brimless velvet hat, soft crown gathered onto wide band. Short leather gloves. Knee-length cloth spats with side-button fastenings; leather shoes with round toes and low heels. 3 7-year-old girl, *c.* 1915. Printed silk party dress with bloused bodice, gathers from under high yoke seam, plain silk collar with lace edge, matching edges on frilled cuffs on long sleeves and edges of frilled two-tier skirt, low waist emphasized by wide velvet belt trimmed with outsized bow on one side, velvet repeated in bands above frilled sleeve cuffs. Large ribbon bow worn in hair on one side. Knitted silk stockings. Leather shoes with bar straps. 4 3-year-old boy, *c.* 1915. Two-piece fine wool suit: short collarless edge-to-edge jacket with long sleeves; knee-length trousers with central creases, wide buttoned waistband and fly fronts. Cotton shirt with buttoned strap fastening, large collar with top-stitched edge, matching cuffs, shirt worn with large silk ribbon bow under collar. Striped knitted cotton socks. Leather boots with side-button fastenings, round toes and low heels. 5 8-year-old girl, *c.* 1915. Knee-length fine wool coat with unfitted wrap-over bodice, large shawl collar trimmed with contrast-colour velvet, matching cuffs on long sleeves and low waist-belt with two button fastening in self-fabric, top-stitched edges and detail. Coat worn over checked cotton dress with square neckline. Felt hat with wide brim and shallow crown trimmed with striped ribbon band. Large ribbon bow worn in hair at back. Short leather gloves. Striped stockings. Long leather boots with side-button fastenings, pointed toes and low heels. 6 3-year-old boy, *c.* 1914. Striped cotton bathing suit: single-breasted blouse, fastening with large buttons, low square neckline and short sleeves; knee-length trousers with buttoned waistband and fly front. Heelless rubber bathing shoes with buttoned bar straps and round toes. 7 6-year-old girl, *c.* 1914. Linen holiday dress, unfitted bodice with buttoned strap fastening under contrast-colour bow, matching colour of trim on large sailor collar, cuffs on three-quarter-length sleeves, hip-level belt and inside of box-pleats on knee-length skirt. Large ribbon bow worn in hair on one side. Long knitted cotton stockings. Leather bar strap shoes with button fastenings, round toes and low heels.

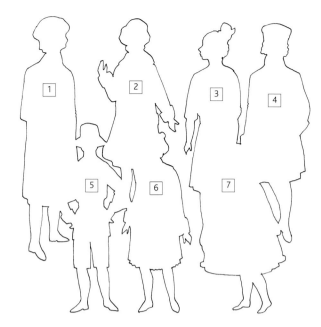

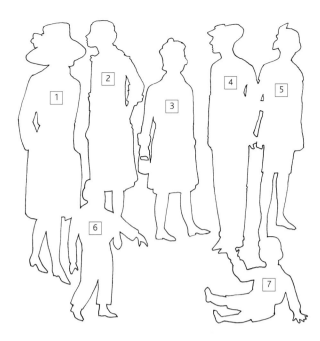

1916–1918

1 9-year-old girl, *c.* 1916. Mid-calf-length rubberized cotton raincoat with offset single-breasted fastening, high collar, long sleeves with buttoned half-strap above wrist level, hip-level patch and flap pockets, top-stitched edges and detail. Rubberized cotton hat with large crown gathered onto close-fitting, turned-down brim. Short leather gloves. Long leather boots with side-button fastenings, pointed toes and low heels. 2 5-year-old girl, *c.* 1918. Knee-length semi-fitted imitation baby lamb coat with buttoned half-belt at back, large contrast-colour imitation fur collar, matching cuffs on long sleeves and trimming around hemline. Felt hat with wide wavy brim and unstructured crown, trimmed with pompons of imitation fur to match trim on coat. Short leather gloves. Woollen stockings. Leather boots with low heels. 3 8-year-old girl, *c.* 1918. Striped wool sleeveless pinafore dress with low square neckline above rows of decorative contrast-fabric-covered buttons, matching button fastenings on each shoulder and on wide waist-belt, knee-length skirt with box pleats sewn to hip level. Striped cotton blouse with centre-front button fastening, stand collar with turned-down top edge and three-quarter-length sleeves gathered into buttoned cuffs. Woollen stockings. Leather bar strap shoes with round toes. 4 8-year-old girl, *c.* 1916. Knee-length single-breasted camel-hair coat with single button fastening under high collar, matching decorative buttons on turned-back cuffs on long sleeves and on hip-level patch pockets, self-fabric belt threaded from inside back through openings in side panel seams and secured by large buckle, top-stitched edges and detail. Brimless cloth hat with tall crown gathered onto narrow band. Woollen stockings. Long leather boots with side-button fastenings and round toes. 5 7-year-old boy, *c.* 1917. Checked wool two-piece suit: hip-length single-breasted collarless jacket, fastening with outsized buttons covered in contrast colour, matching colour of wide belt and buttons and three shaped flap pockets; knee-length trousers with fly fronts. Cotton shirt with large collar and turned-back buttoned cuffs, shirt worn with large pleated silk bow tie. Checked wool hat with wide turned-down brim and high crown with contrast-colour band, fabrics matching suit. Knee-length woollen socks. Lace-up leather shoes with round toes and low heels. 6 6-year-old girl, *c.* 1916. Knee-length unfitted imitation fur coat, double-breasted fastening with outsized buttons from under large collar, long sleeves with deep cuffs. Coat worn over cotton dress with knife-pleat hemline. Brimless knitted wool beret with large unstructured crown gathered onto narrow band. Long woollen stockings. Short leather boots with side-button fastenings, round toes and low heels. 7 5-year-old girl, *c.* 1918. Knee-length wool coat, flared from shoulders to hems of fur-trimmed skirts, matching fur collar, fur concealing side-button fastening and trim on hems of long raglan-style sleeves, buckled self-fabric belt threaded from inside back through openings on side fronts. Felt hat with wide turned-down brim and shallow crown trimmed with band of fur to match coat trimming. Long leather boots with side-button fastenings, round toes and low heels.

1919–1920

1 12-year-old girl, *c.* 1920. Single-breasted checked wool tweed coat, worn open and held with buttoned waist-belt, collar with long revers, full-length sleeves, large hip-level patch pockets with button trim, matching coat fastenings. Knee-length patterned cotton dress with low frill-edged neckline. Straw hat, wide brim lined with coloured silk, tall crown trimmed with diagonal ribbon and artificial cherries. Large ribbon bow worn in hair at back. Pale-coloured silk stockings. Leather shoes with ribbon laces, pointed toes and high heels. 2 9-year-old girl, *c.* 1919. Knee-length floral-patterned cotton dress, bloused bodice with asymmetric button fastening under shoulder-wide plain contrast-colour collar with rouleau bow trim and double frilled edge, matching detail on cuffs on elbow-length sleeves, large hip-level patch pockets in full skirt and colour of wide waist-sash. Ribbon worn low on forehead and tied in bow on one side. Pale-coloured stockings. Leather shoes with buckle trim above pointed toes. 3 7-year-old girl, *c.* 1920. Single-breasted fine wool coat, fastening with outsized buttons under fur collar, matching cuffs on long sleeves and trim on hip-level patch pockets in full skirts, long self-fabric belt buttoned on each side front, crossed over on centre front and buttoned to top of pockets. Brimless fur hat with pompon trim on top of high crown. Short leather gloves. Small leather handbag with short handle. Woollen stockings. Long leather boots with side-button fastenings, pointed toes and low heels. 4 12-year-old boy, *c.* 1919. Two-piece wool flannel suit: single-breasted jacket with two button fastening above high waist seam, collar with wide revers, single breast pocket and hip-length jetted pockets in skirts, top-stitched edges and detail; narrow ankle-length trousers with central creases and turn-ups. Cotton shirt with attached collar, worn with silk necktie. Wool cap with full crown and large peak. Leather lace-up shoes with pointed toes and low heels. 5 9-year-old girl, *c.* 1920. Two-piece striped cotton bathing costume: long loose-fitting top fastening with single button on each shoulder above low V-shaped neckline, edged with plain contrast-colour cotton, matching cuffs on short sleeves, hem and side vents of skirt, hems of short drawers and buttoned hip-level belt. Spotted cotton turban-style hat with knotted bow on one side. Heelless rubber bathing shoes with ribbon fastening and round toes. 6 4-year-old boy, *c.* 1920. One-piece cotton playsuit with contrast-colour buttoned strap fastening, matching colour of bound edges of large Peter Pan collar, inset waist-belt and tops of hip-level patch pockets, long sleeves with sewn cuffs piped with second contrast colour, repeated above hems of ankle-length trousers and all other edges and seams. Leather sandals with buckled strap fastenings, open detail, round toes and low heels. 7 2-year-old boy, *c.* 1919. Striped cotton shirt with bloused bodice, long sleeves gathered into cuffs at wrist level, large collar worn with patterned necktie, blouse buttoned at waist level to shorts, three-button trim on outside leg seam above hems. Cotton canvas hat with large turned-back brim edged with coloured braid, matching trim on sections of large crown. Ankle-length cotton socks with patterned edge. Heelless cloth shoes with buttoned bar straps, round toes and leather soles.

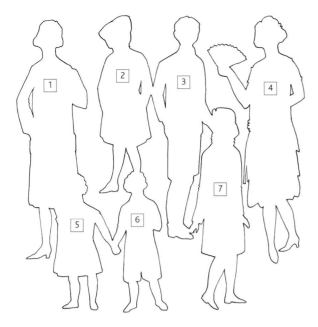

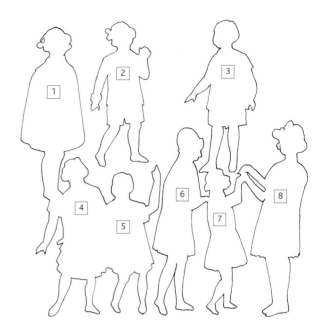

1921–1923

1 12-year-old girl, *c.* 1923. Knee-length cotton dress with hip-length unfitted bodice, V-shaped neckline with contrast-colour collar, matching cuffs on full-length sleeves, hip-level belt and covered buttons of asymmetric side fastening, ribbon flower and ends under centre point of neckline, matching colour of button on belt, straight skirt. Flesh-coloured silk stockings. Leather bar strap shoes with pointed toes and high heels. 2 4-year-old boy, *c.* 1921. Single-breasted ribbed cotton velvet coat with plain contrast-colour cotton velvet collar, matching hip-level flap pockets and covered buttons. Cotton hat with turned-down brim, high crown cut in sections and self-covered button trim on centre top. Long knitted wool socks. Leather bar strap shoes with round toes and low heels. 3 8-year-old boy, *c.* 1922. Knitted wool shirt with small collar, buttoned strap fastening and full-length sleeves with buttoned cuffs. Knee-length wool trousers with central creases and fly fronts. Knee-length knitted wool socks with patterned turned-down cuffs. Lace-up leather ankle boots with rounded toecaps and low heels. 4 12-year-old girl, *c.* 1923. Silk party dress, hip-length unfitted bodice with wide round neckline edged with pleated frill, matching hems of short sleeves, multicoloured ribbon flowers and ends on one side hip, above scalloped tiers of knee-length skirt. Multicoloured ribbon flowers worn as hair decoration on one side of head, matching dress trimming. Flesh-coloured silk stockings. Leather shoes with buttoned bar straps, pointed toes and high heels. 5 3-year-old girl, *c.* 1922. Cotton dress with wide round neckline, cap sleeves and knee-length flared skirt, patterned cotton panels from chest level to above skirt hemline, scalloped at top and bottom and edged in contrast colour, matching narrow belt decorated with tiny rosettes. Short knitted cotton socks. Heelless leather shoes with buttoned bar straps and round toes. 6 3-year-old boy, *c.* 1921. Two-piece cotton suit: double-breasted jacket, fastening with pearl buttons, large pointed collar bound with contrast colour, matching attached buttoned waist-belt, sewn cuffs on long sleeves and button-trimmed side panels above hems of knee-length trousers. Long knitted cotton socks with patterned top edges. Heelless leather pumps with low-cut fronts and round toes. 7 8-year-old girl, *c.* 1922. Woollen school coat, single-breasted, fastening with large buttons, wide buttonable revers and large collar, long sleeves with top-stitched sewn cuffs, matching edges of hip-level patch and flap pockets and buttoned waist-belt. Felt hat with wide turned-down brim and large crown with draped band and large bow trim on one side. Short leather gloves. Dark knitted cotton stockings. Leather shoes with ribbon laces, pointed toecaps and low heels.

1924–1925

1 4-year-old girl, *c.* 1925. Knee-length faux fur cape, single-breasted fastening with large self-fabric covered buttons, high neckline with large collar, waist-level vertical opening on either side of centre front. Faux fur hat with padded brim and pompon suspended on cord from centre of high crown. Faux fur hand muff. Cape worn over wool jacket with long sleeves. Knee-length knitted cotton socks. Leather shoes with buttoned bar straps, round toes and low heels. 2 2-year-old boy, *c.* 1924. Knitted wool two-piece playsuit: hip-length top with buttoned fastening under high square neckline to chest level, shaped yoke outlined with contrast colour, matching cuffs on long sleeves and hems of top and shorts. Knitted wool hat with turned-back brim edged with contrast colour, matching pompons on side of high crown. Ankle-length knitted cotton socks. Leather shoes with buttoned ankle straps, round toes and low heels. 3 3-year-old boy, *c.* 1924. Two-piece linen playsuit: long unfitted top with hip-level top-stitched tuck, large collar edged with contrast colour, matching short buttoned strap fastening, hems of short sleeves, tops of patch pockets with button trim and knee-length shorts with centre-front creases. Long knitted cotton socks with patterned turned-down cuffs. Leather shoes with buttoned bar straps, round toes and low heels. 4 5-year-old girl, *c.* 1925. Sleeveless cotton dress, cape collar with appliqué flower motifs in each corner and contrast-colour bound edges, matching piping on wide neckline, edges of top two tiers of three-tier skirt and bow trim on side hip. Knee-length knitted cotton socks. Leather shoes with buttoned ankle straps, low heels and bow trim above round toes. 5 3-year-old boy, *c.* 1925. Two-piece cotton playsuit: long flared top, high round neckline with top-stitched edge, matching hems of short sleeves, off-centre button strap fastening above two knife pleats and hem facings decorated with appliqué birds and trees; shorts gathered into knee-level bands with button fastenings. Short knitted cotton socks. Heelless leather shoes with buttoned bar straps and round toes. 6 6-year-old girl, *c.* 1924. Cotton dress with hip-length single-breasted unfitted bodice, fastening with contrast-colour covered buttons, matching edges of scalloped collar, scalloped cuffs on long sleeves, buckled belt and inside facings of box-pleats in knee-length skirt, pleats decorated with appliqué fabric flowers and leaves above hemline. Felt hat with turned-back contrast-colour brim bound with coloured ribbon and sectioned crown decorated at the back with appliqué felt flowers and leaves. Knee-length knitted cotton socks. Leather shoes with buttoned bar straps, round toes and low heels. 7 4-year-old girl, *c.* 1924. Patterned cotton dress, unfitted bodice trimmed with contrast-colour covered buttons on centre front, matching edge of collar, band of short puff sleeves above pleated hem and on patch pockets on short gathered skirt. Short knitted cotton socks. Leather shoes with buttoned bar straps, low heels and round toes. 8 6-year-old girl, *c.* 1924. Spotted silk party dress with high collarless neckline, trimmed on centre front with self-fabric bow and long ends, matching trim on belt under hip-length bloused bodice, pleats repeated on hems of short sleeves, decorative apron front and hemline of knee-length skirt. Large bow worn in hair on one side. Knee-length knitted cotton socks. Satin pumps with low heels and bow trim above round toes.

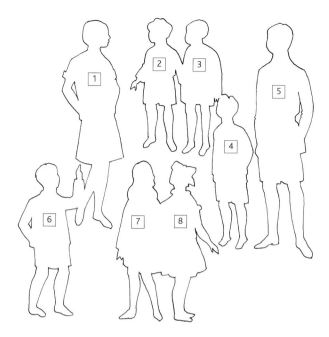

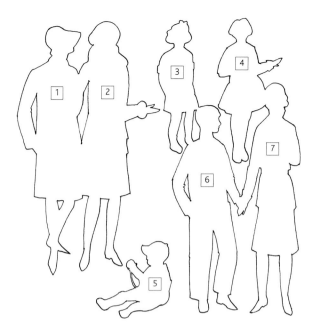

1926–1928

1 8-year-old girl, c. 1926. Checked wool dress, long unfitted bloused bodice with chest-level V-shaped yoke, plain cotton collar and matching cuffs on short sleeves, black satin bow worn under collar, matching narrow bucked hip-level belt above knee-length box-pleated skirt. Cotton stockings. Leather shoes with buttoned bar straps, round toes and low heels.

2 2-year-old boy, c. 1928. Cotton blouse, large collar above buttoned strap fastening with rows of pin-tucks on either side, long sleeves gathered into cuffs. Knee-length cotton shorts with wide buttoned-on braces, front zip fastening and centre-front creases. Knitted cotton ankle socks. Heelless leather shoes with buttoned bar straps and round toes. 3 2-year-old boy, c. 1926. Two-piece linen suit: long top with contrast-colour asymmetric mock collar, matching large button trim above hemline under collar and trim on single chest-level patch pocket, detachable plain cotton collar and cuffs on long sleeves; shorts with centre-front creases. Long knitted cotton socks. Leather shoes, T-straps with buckle fastenings, round toes and low heels. 4 3-year-old boy, c. 1928. Two-piece wool suit: long top with hip-level top-stitched tuck under two jetted pockets, long sleeves, large collar above wide strap fastening with outsized pearl buttons, coloured silk scarf worn inside collar and threaded through open hem of strap fastening; shorts with centre-front creases. Long knitted cotton socks. Leather shoes, T-straps with buckle fastenings, round toes and low heels. 5 8-year-old boy, c. 1927. Two-piece wool tweed suit: long single-breasted jacket with tie belt, two hip-level patch pockets and single breast pocket, long sleeves with stitched cuffs; knee-length trousers with centre-front creases. Cotton shirt, attached collar with top-stitched edges, worn open. Long knitted wool socks with turned-down cuffs. Lace-up leather shoes with round toecaps and low heels. 6 4-year-old boy, c. 1927. Two-piece velvet suit: collarless edge-to-edge jacket with long sleeves; shorts with centre-front creases. Satin blouse with large ruffle-edged collar, matching edges of buttoned strap fastening. Long knitted cotton socks. Leather shoes with buttoned bar straps, round toes and low heels. 7 5-year-old girl, c. 1928. Unfitted double-breasted wool coat, fastening with large self-fabric covered buttons, long sleeves and hip-level decorative seam, coat worn with miniature fox fur stole around neck. Felt hat with turned-down brim, tall crown decorated with contrast-colour band and felt appliqué flower on front. Short leather gloves. Woollen stockings. Canvas spats with side-button fastenings, leather shoes with round toes and low heels. 8 5-year-old girl, c. 1926. Velvet dress with bloused bodice gathered from under fur-trimmed neckline, fur repeated on hems of short sleeves, hip-level belt fastened on one side with self-fabric covered button above knee-length gathered skirt. Large ribbon bow worn in hair on one side. Long knitted cotton socks. Leather shoes, bar straps with button fastenings, round toes and low heels.

1929–1930

1 10-year-old girl, c. 1929. Speckled wool tweed coat, small collar with long narrow revers to side hip above single button fastening, panel seams running diagonally from under arms through unfitted bodice and vertically from low waist level through straight knee-length skirts to hemline, hip-level patch pockets with buttoned strap detail, matching detail above hems of long sleeves. Silk blouse, Peter Pan collar and front button fastening with pin-tucked detail on either side. Felt hat with wide turned-down brim at front, narrowing to back, domed crown with contrast-colour petersham band. Short leather gloves. Knee-length knitted stockings. Leather shoes with buttoned bar straps, pointed toes and low heels. 2 12-year-old girl, c. 1929. Wool coat with single button fastening on side hip under long top-stitched satin-faced revers, matching front edge facings and two flap pockets on either side at hip level above flared asymmetric panels, large fur collar with matching cuffs on long sleeves. Masculine-style shirt with attached contrast-colour collar, worn with silk necktie. Close-fitting felt hat with narrow turned-down brim and domed crown trimmed with appliqué leaves on one side. Short leather gloves. Silk stockings. Leather shoes with wide buttoned bar straps, pointed toes and low heels. 3 2-year-old girl, c. 1930. Hip-length unfitted cotton blouse with patterned contrast-colour collar, matching turned-back cuffs on short sleeves. Above-knee-length short flared skirt in fabric to match blouse. Hair band with bow on front. Short knitted cotton socks. Heelless leather shoes with buttoned bar straps and round toes.

4 3-year-old girl, c. 1930. Patterned cotton dress with unfitted bodice and gathered knee-length skirt, plain cotton Peter Pan collar, matching stiffened front panel with self-fabric covered button fastening and turned-back cuffs on long sleeves, dress worn with narrow leather belt on hipline. Short knitted cotton socks. Leather shoes with T-straps and round toes.

5 18-month-old boy, c. 1929. Two-piece cotton playsuit: bodice with Peter Pan collar edged in narrow lace and embroidered with flowers and leaves, matching cuffs on short puff sleeves, embroidered emblem on centre front and waistband with buttons, attaching full knickers to top, buttoned gusset between elasticated legs. Fine cotton bonnet with embroidered frilled brim, full gathered crown and ribbon fastenings under chin. Short knitted cotton socks. Heelless cloth shoes, two bar straps with button fastenings and round toes. 6 8-year-old boy, c. 1929. One-piece heavy-duty cotton playsuit, long sleeves with top-stitched cuffs, matching edges of pointed collar, crotch-length buttoned strap fastening, inset waistband, chest-level buttoned patch pockets, hip-level patch and flap pockets, seams, details and hems of wide ankle-length trousers. Leather shoes with laced fastenings, round toecaps and low heels. 7 9-year-old girl, c. 1930. Two-piece wool jersey suit: hip-length single-breasted jacket with self-fabric covered buttons from neck to hem, scallop-edged collar, matching turned-back cuffs on long sleeves, piped pockets above and below buttoned waist-belt; knee-length flared skirt. Pull-on knitted wool hat with turned-back brim and soft crown. Knee-length knitted wool socks. Leather shoes with buttoned bar straps, pointed toes and low heels.

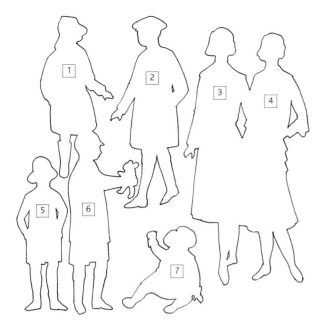

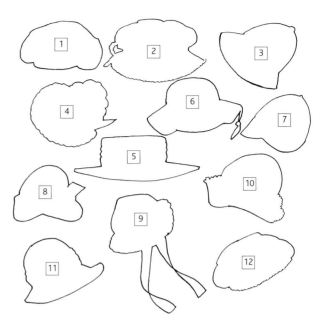

1931–1933

1 4-year-old girl, *c.* 1933. Waterproofed cotton raincoat with double-breasted fastening under small pointed collar, long raglan-style sleeves with buttoned strap above wrists, diagonal welt pockets at hip level in flared skirts, wide buckled belt, top-stitched edges and detail. Waterproofed cotton sou'wester-style hat with turned-down brim, longer at back than front, sectioned crown, top-stitched edges and detail. Knee-length rubber boots. 2 7-year-old boy, *c.* 1932. Double-breasted knee-length wool tweed coat with flat collar and wide revers, long sleeves with two button trim above hem, single breast pocket, diagonal hip-length pockets. Cotton shirt with attached collar, worn with silk necktie. Wool tweed peaked cap with large soft crown. Knee-length knitted wool socks, turned-down cuffs with contrast-colour pattern. Leather shoes with laced fastenings, round toecaps and low heels. 3 12-year-old girl, *c.* 1933. Sleeveless wool pinafore dress with low pointed square neckline above double-breasted fastening with square novelty buttons, matching inset waistband, knee-length flared skirt with box-pleats, top-stitched edges and detail. Checked cotton blouse with shirt-style collar above keyhole opening bound with contrast-colour velvet, matching rouleau bow fastenings, keyhole and bow repeated at wrist level on long full sleeves. Silk stockings. Leather shoes with buttoned bar straps, pointed toes and low heels. 4 12-year-old girl, *c.* 1933. Silk party dress, bloused bodice with frill-edged collar, repeated on hems of long sleeves, three tiers of spotted silk chiffon from waist to hip level, matching elbow-level frill on sleeves and overlay on collar, knee-length flared skirt, contrast-colour velvet belt with cut steel buckle, velvet repeated in covered button trim above sleeve hems. Silk stockings. Satin pumps with low-cut fronts, pointed toes and low heels. 5 4-year-old boy, *c.* 1931. Striped cotton sun suit, bib front with buttoned straps, inset waistband, knee-length shorts with hip-level patch pockets and front zip opening. Stiffened striped cotton hat, turned-down brim with contrast-colour lining, high crown and inset band. Short knitted cotton socks. Leather sandals, T-straps with buckle fastenings, round toes and low heels. 6 7-year-old boy, *c.* 1931. Double-breasted striped wool jacket, fastening with brass buttons, matching trim at wrist level on long sleeves, hip-level patch pockets, collar and revers edged with coloured braid. Wool flannel shorts with central creases. Peaked wool cap with close-fitting sectioned crown, button trim on top. Knee-length knitted wool socks, turned-down cuffs with coloured pattern. Leather shoes with laced fastenings, round toecaps and low heels. 7 18-month-old girl, *c.* 1933. Single-breasted fine wool coat, scalloped frill-edged and embroidered collar trimmed with ribbon, matching turned-back cuffs on long sleeves, skirts gathered from high round yoke. Silk bonnet, frilled brim lined with contrast colour, full gathered crown and silk ribbon ties. Short knitted cotton socks. Heelless cloth shoes with buttoned bar straps and round toes.

Hats 1917–1933

1 12-year-old girl, *c.* 1917. Velvet beret with full crown, falling to one side and gathered onto wide band, embroidered with garlands of multicoloured leaves and flowers, silk lining. 2 12-year-old girl, *c.* 1920. Silk hat with large unstructured crown, gathered onto turned-down wired brim covered with ruched self-fabric and edged with gold braid, matching narrow band, wired bow and ends. 3 6-year-old boy, *c.* 1917. Stiffened cotton hat with tall crown cut in sections, self-fabric covered button on top, wide inset band above turned-down wired brim, top-stitched edges and detail, leather inner band and silk lining. 4 4-year-old girl, *c.* 1923. Fine silk velvet hat, tall crown ruched between three rows of narrow inset contrast-colour satin piping, matching covered button on top and bow with long ends on one side of ruched and padded brim. 5 10-year-old girl, *c.* 1921. Stiffened straw hat with tall flat-topped crown, wide striped silk band and wide flat brim, leather inner band. 6 6-year-old girl, *c.* 1924. Stiffened cotton hat with tall crown cut in sections, wide turned-up brim decorated across the front with brightly coloured appliqué flowers and leaves, leather inner band, cord and tassel trim on one side. 7 10-year-old boy, *c.* 1932. Wool cap with small stiffened peak, close-fitting crown cut in sections and piped with cord, school badge on centre front and self-fabric covered button on top, self-fabric inner band and cotton lining. 8 4-year-old boy, *c.* 1918. Stiffened cotton hat, tall crown cut in two pieces, saddle-stitching on either side seam, matching edges of wide contrast-colour band and ends and turned-up brim. 9 4-year-old girl, *c.* 1927. Velvet hat with pointed and ruched crown attached to wide self-fabric ruched band above wide padded fur brim trimmed with wax flowers and leaves on one side, long velvet ribbons to tie under chin. 10 5-year-old girl, *c.* 1925. Felt hat with wide brim turned up in front of close-fitting crown and down at sides and back, edges trimmed with box-pleated silk ribbon, three coloured pompons decorating one side towards back. 11 12-year-old girl, *c.* 1928. Stiffened felt hat with tall dome-shaped crown with wide draped silk band, wide brim, turned down at back and front edge turned up from sides. 12 10-year-old girl, *c.* 1933. Silk beret with full crown gathered onto narrow band threaded with elastic, self-fabric lining.

Hats 1934–1950

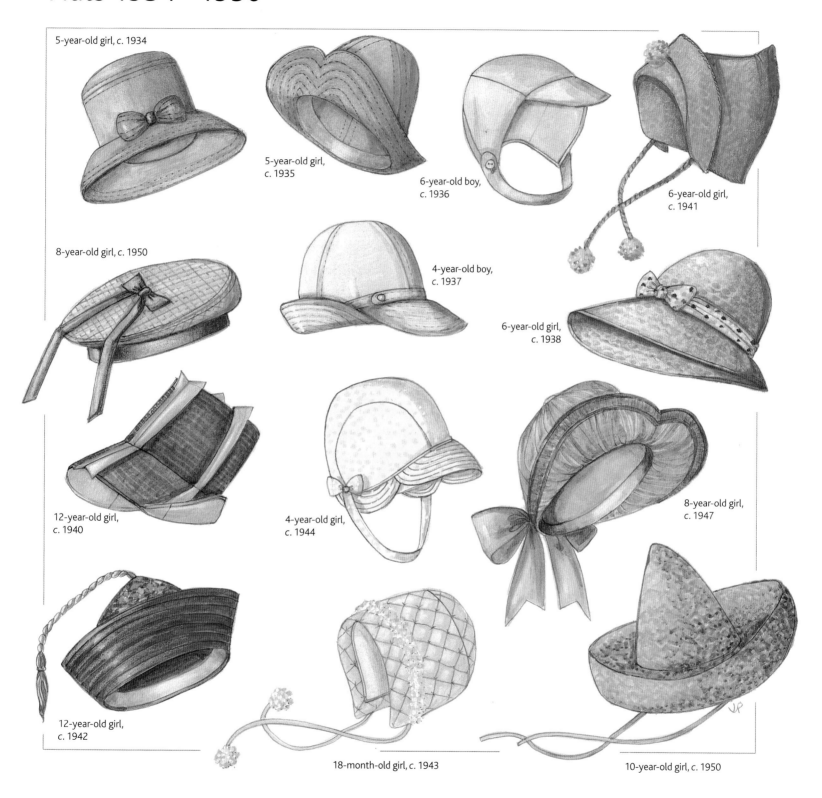

5-year-old girl, c. 1934

5-year-old girl, c. 1935

6-year-old boy, c. 1936

6-year-old girl, c. 1941

8-year-old girl, c. 1950

4-year-old boy, c. 1937

6-year-old girl, c. 1938

12-year-old girl, c. 1940

4-year-old girl, c. 1944

8-year-old girl, c. 1947

12-year-old girl, c. 1942

18-month-old girl, c. 1943

10-year-old girl, c. 1950

1934–1935

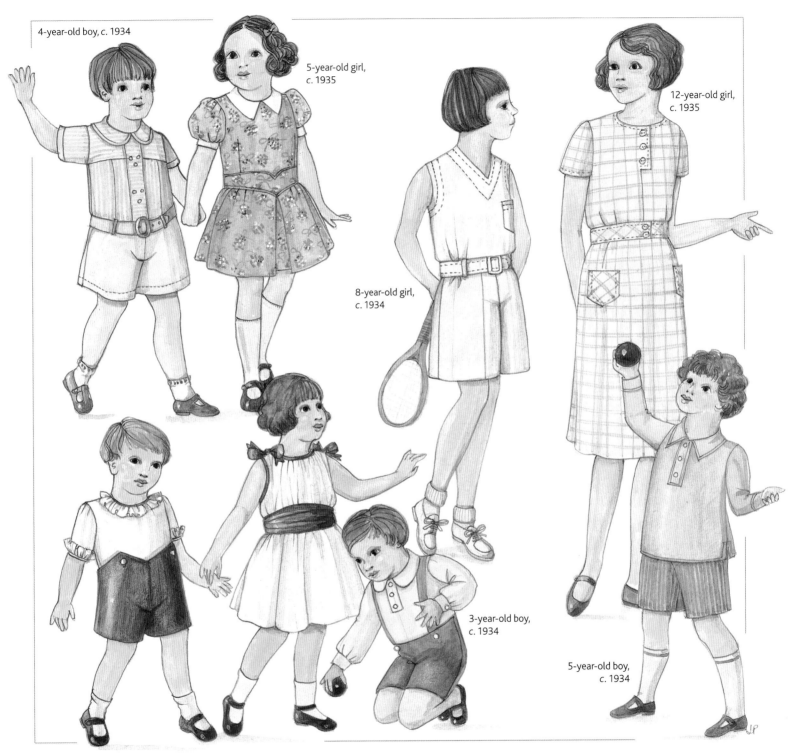

4-year-old boy, *c.* 1934

5-year-old girl, *c.* 1935

8-year-old girl, *c.* 1934

12-year-old girl, *c.* 1935

3-year-old boy, *c.* 1934

5-year-old boy, *c.* 1934

3-year-old boy, *c.* 1935

5-year-old girl, *c.* 1935

1936 – 1938

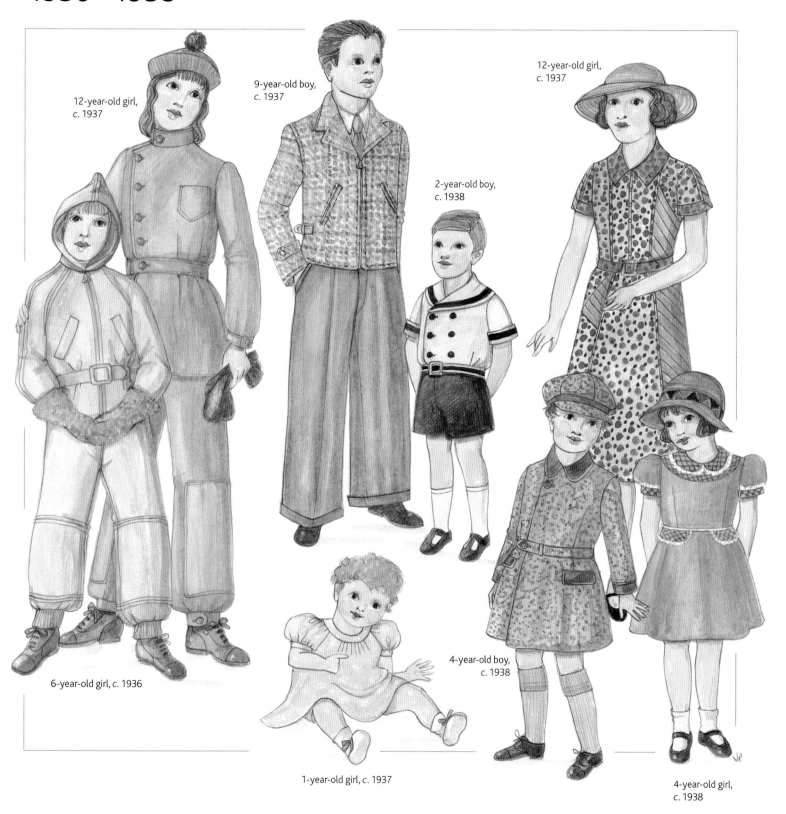

12-year-old girl,
c. 1937

9-year-old boy,
c. 1937

12-year-old girl,
c. 1937

2-year-old boy,
c. 1938

6-year-old girl, c. 1936

1-year-old girl, c. 1937

4-year-old boy,
c. 1938

4-year-old girl,
c. 1938

1939 – 1940

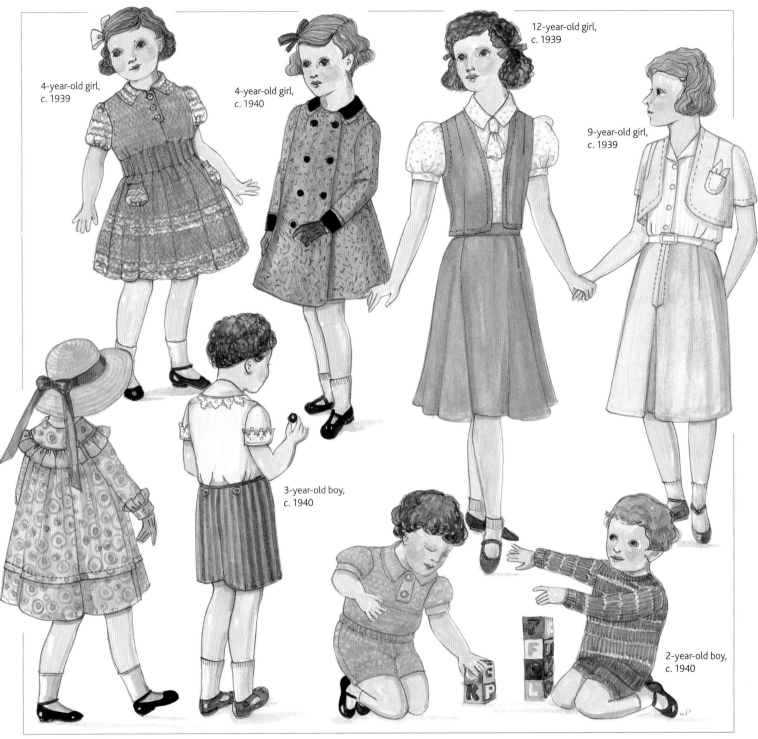

4-year-old girl, c. 1939

4-year-old girl, c. 1940

12-year-old girl, c. 1939

9-year-old girl, c. 1939

3-year-old boy, c. 1940

2-year-old boy, c. 1940

3-year-old girl, c. 1939

2-year-old boy, c. 1940

1941–1942

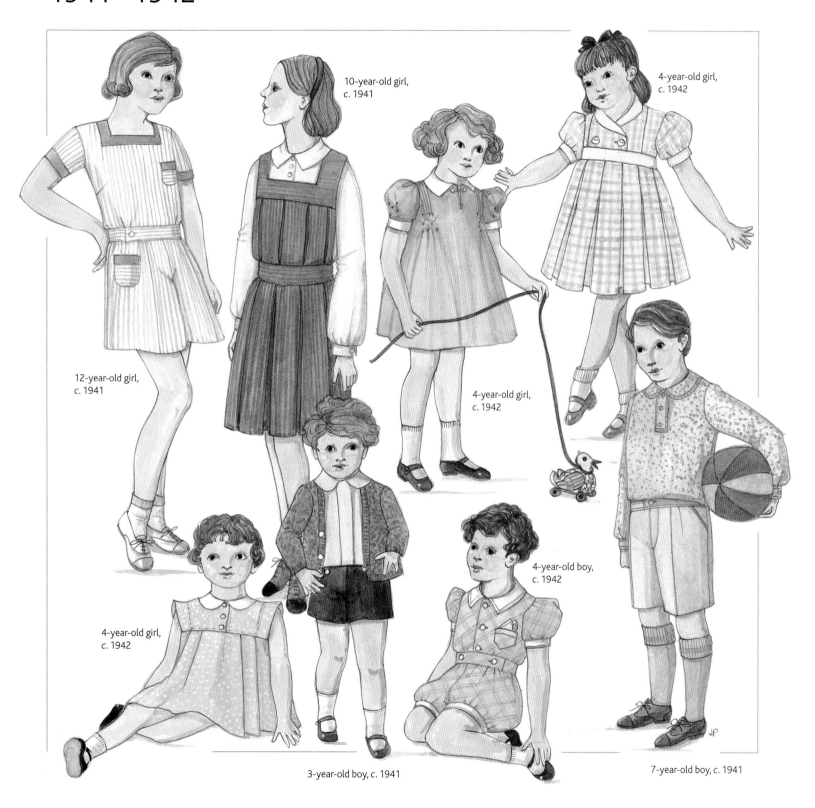

10-year-old girl,
c. 1941

4-year-old girl,
c. 1942

12-year-old girl,
c. 1941

4-year-old girl,
c. 1942

4-year-old girl,
c. 1942

4-year-old boy,
c. 1942

3-year-old boy, c. 1941

7-year-old boy, c. 1941

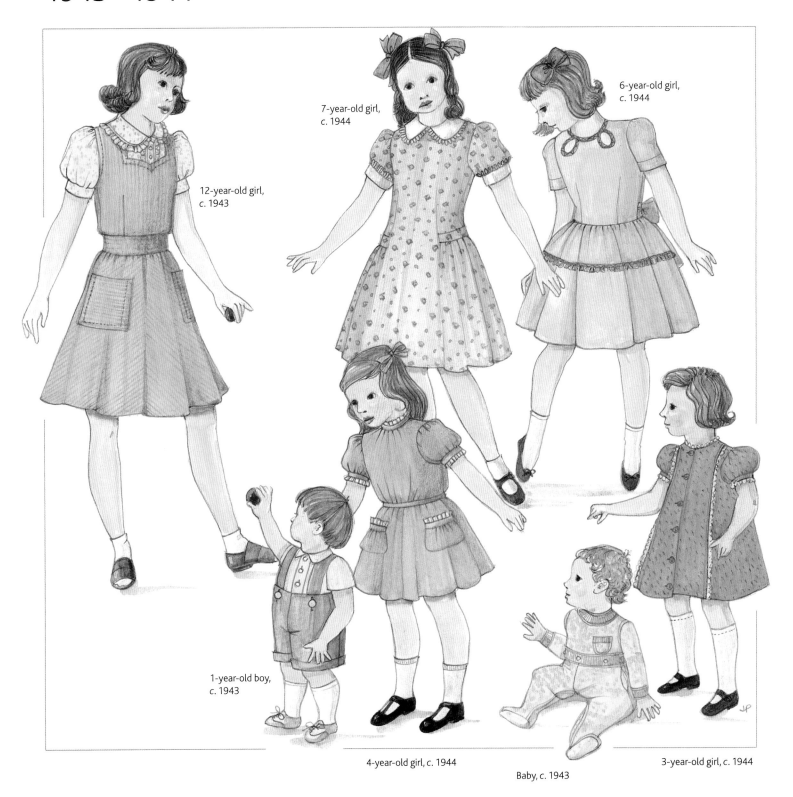

12-year-old girl,
c. 1943

7-year-old girl,
c. 1944

6-year-old girl,
c. 1944

1-year-old boy,
c. 1943

4-year-old girl, c. 1944

Baby, c. 1943

3-year-old girl, c. 1944

1945–1946

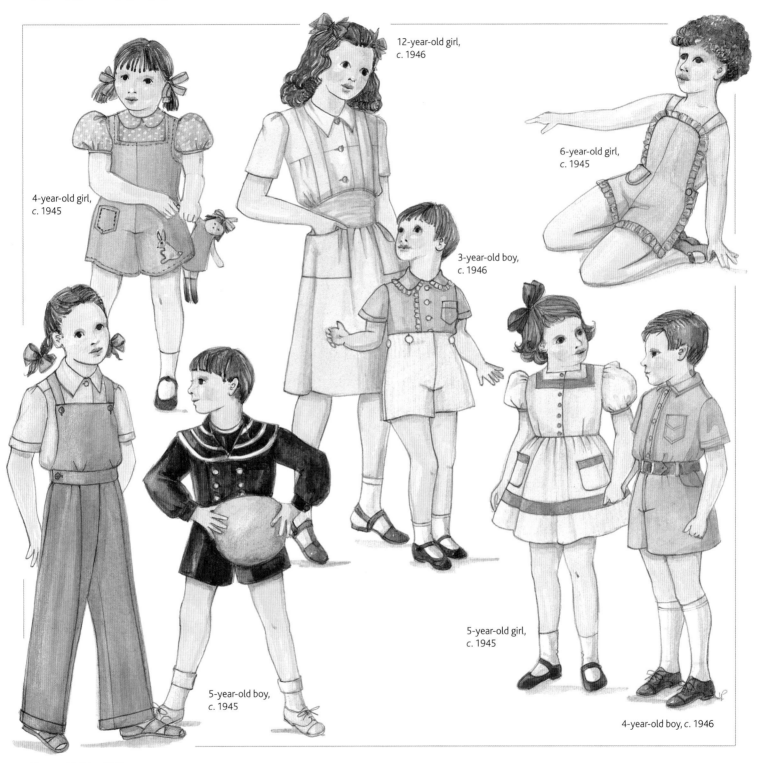

12-year-old girl, c. 1946

6-year-old girl, c. 1945

4-year-old girl, c. 1945

3-year-old boy, c. 1946

5-year-old boy, c. 1945

5-year-old girl, c. 1945

4-year-old boy, c. 1946

7-year-old girl, c. 1946

1947–1948

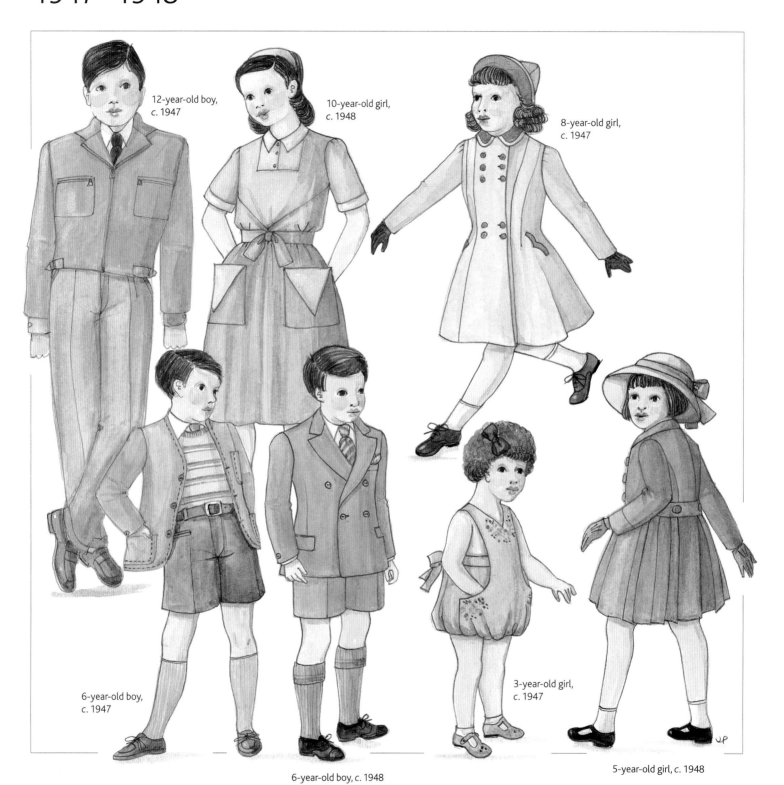

12-year-old boy, *c.* 1947

10-year-old girl, *c.* 1948

8-year-old girl, *c.* 1947

6-year-old boy, *c.* 1947

6-year-old boy, *c.* 1948

3-year-old girl, *c.* 1947

5-year-old girl, *c.* 1948

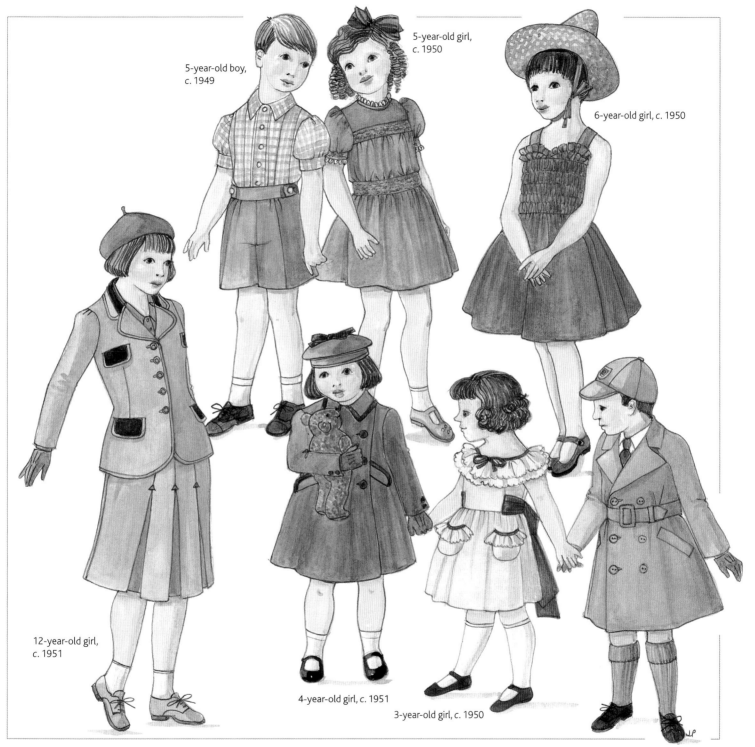

5-year-old boy,
c. 1949

5-year-old girl,
c. 1950

6-year-old girl, c. 1950

12-year-old girl,
c. 1951

4-year-old girl, c. 1951

3-year-old girl, c. 1950

5-year-old boy, c. 1951

1952–1953

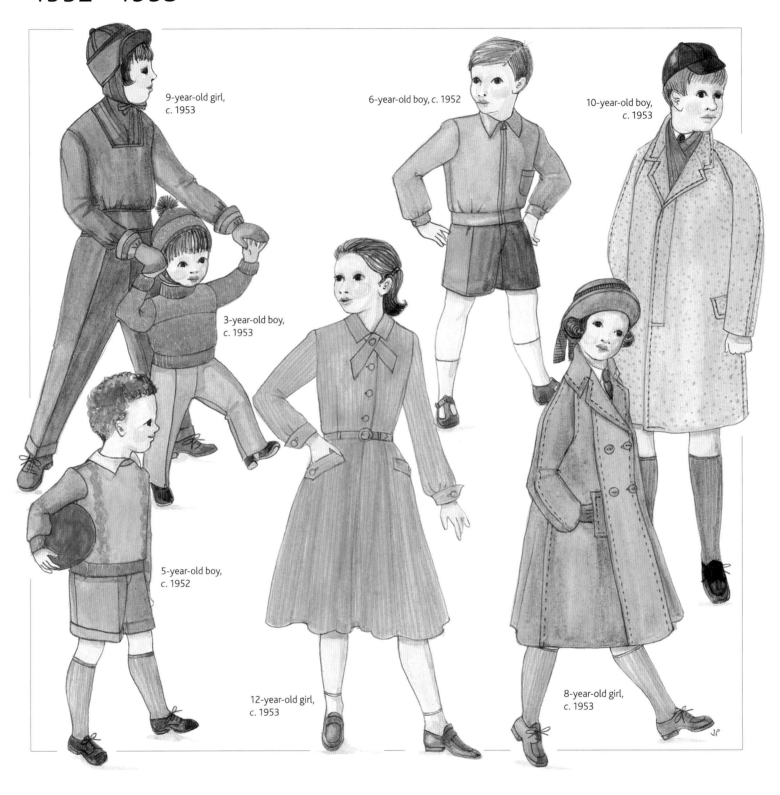

9-year-old girl, *c.* 1953

6-year-old boy, *c.* 1952

10-year-old boy, *c.* 1953

3-year-old boy, *c.* 1953

5-year-old boy, *c.* 1952

12-year-old girl, *c.* 1953

8-year-old girl, *c.* 1953

1954–1956

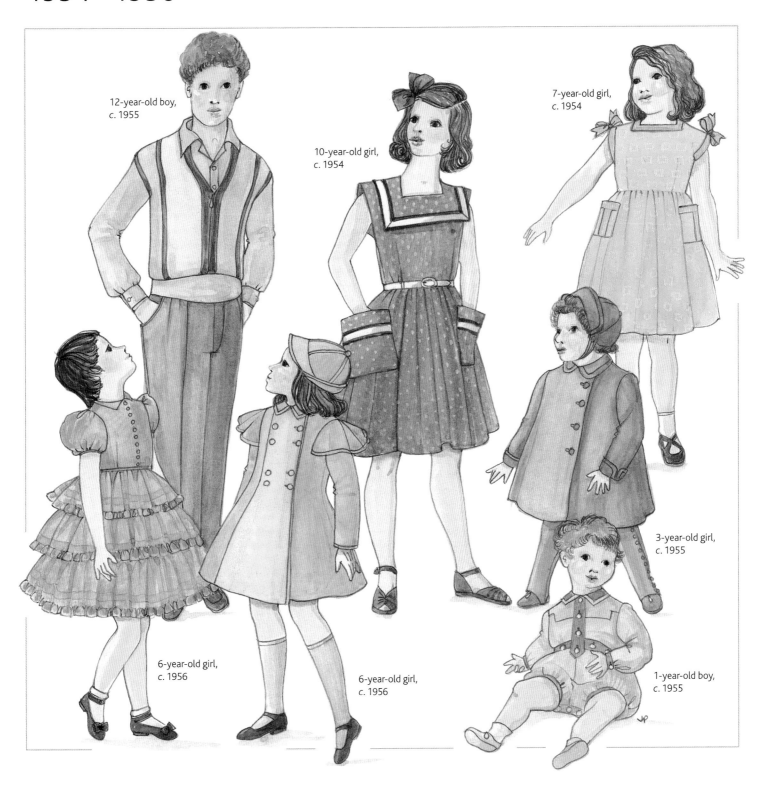

12-year-old boy,
c. 1955

10-year-old girl,
c. 1954

7-year-old girl,
c. 1954

6-year-old girl,
c. 1956

6-year-old girl,
c. 1956

3-year-old girl,
c. 1955

1-year-old boy,
c. 1955

1957–1958

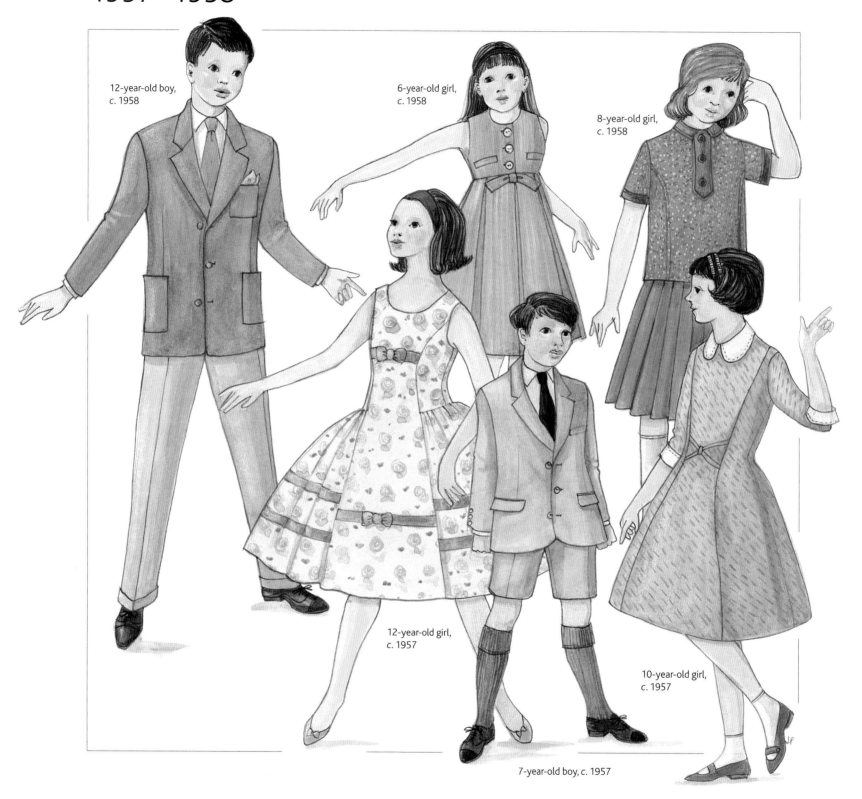

12-year-old boy, *c.* 1958

6-year-old girl, *c.* 1958

8-year-old girl, *c.* 1958

12-year-old girl, *c.* 1957

7-year-old boy, *c.* 1957

10-year-old girl, *c.* 1957

1959–1961

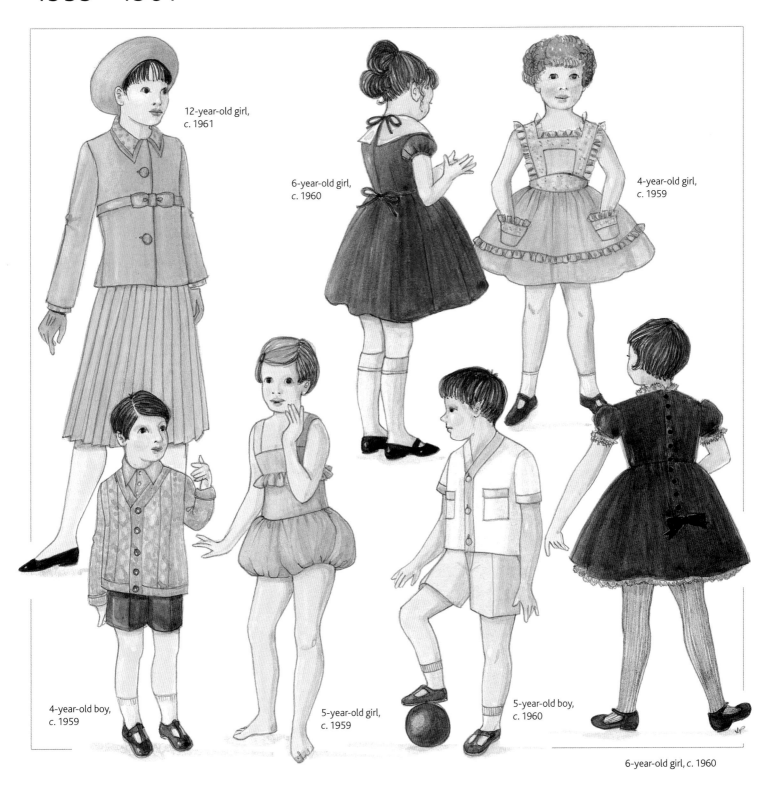

12-year-old girl, *c.* 1961

6-year-old girl, *c.* 1960

4-year-old girl, *c.* 1959

4-year-old boy, *c.* 1959

5-year-old girl, *c.* 1959

5-year-old boy, *c.* 1960

6-year-old girl, *c.* 1960

1962 –1963

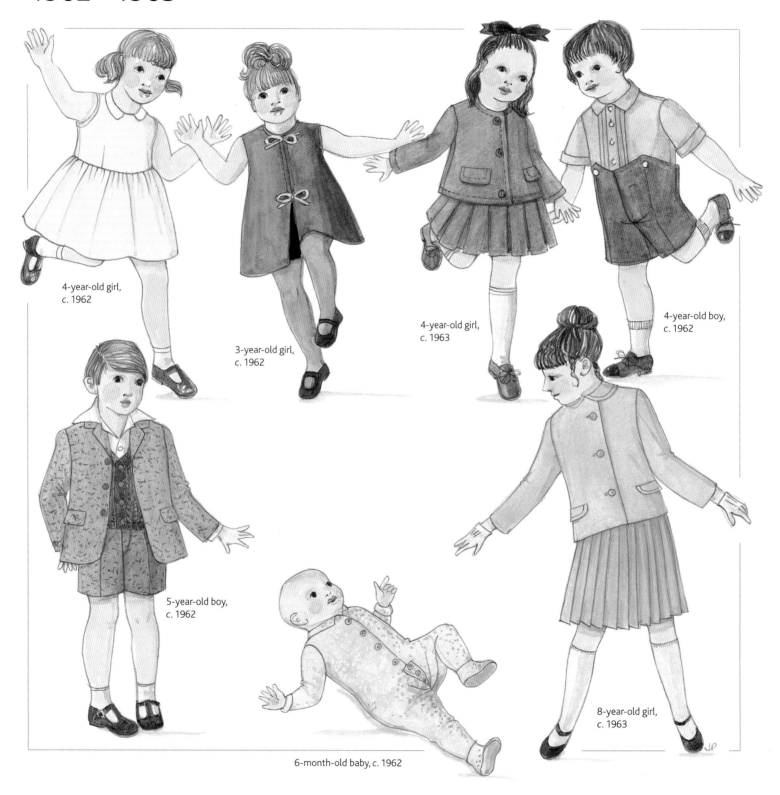

4-year-old girl,
c. 1962

3-year-old girl,
c. 1962

4-year-old girl,
c. 1963

4-year-old boy,
c. 1962

5-year-old boy,
c. 1962

6-month-old baby, c. 1962

8-year-old girl,
c. 1963

1964–1966

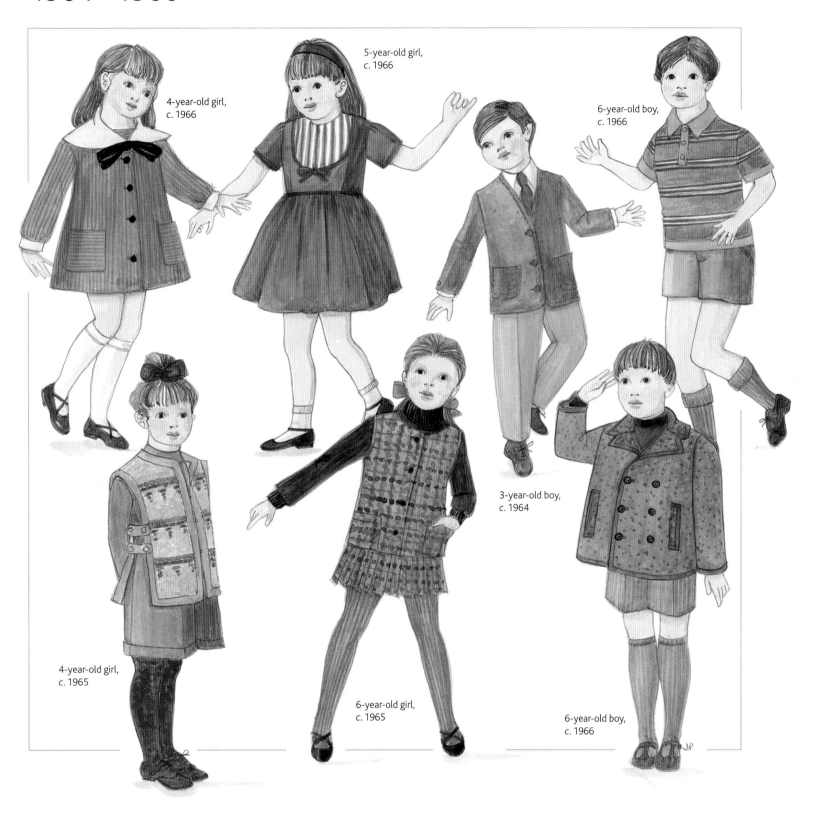

4-year-old girl,
c. 1966

5-year-old girl,
c. 1966

6-year-old boy,
c. 1966

4-year-old girl,
c. 1965

3-year-old boy,
c. 1964

6-year-old girl,
c. 1965

6-year-old boy,
c. 1966

Accessories 1951–1966

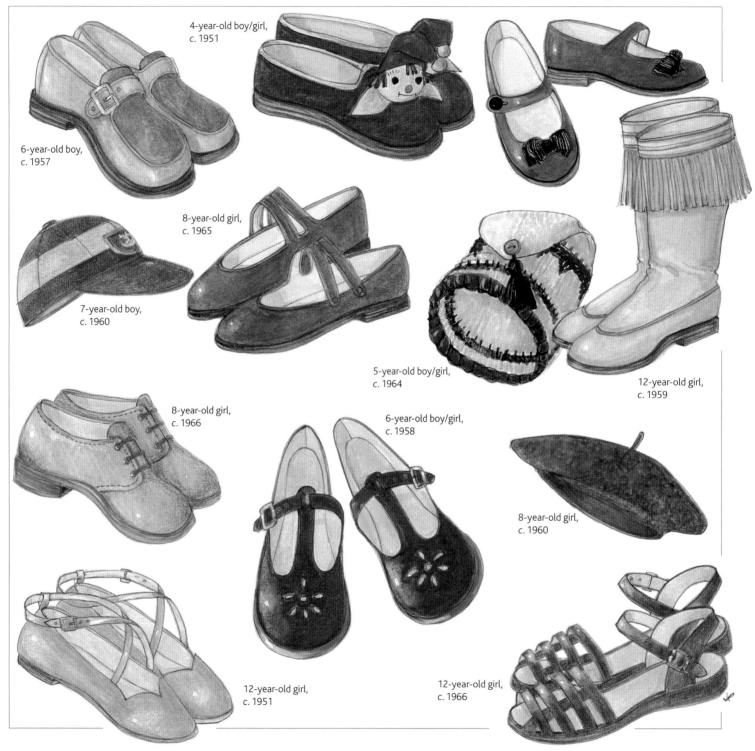

4-year-old boy/girl,
c. 1951

5-year-old girl, c. 1952

6-year-old boy,
c. 1957

8-year-old girl,
c. 1965

7-year-old boy,
c. 1960

5-year-old boy/girl,
c. 1964

12-year-old girl,
c. 1959

8-year-old girl,
c. 1966

6-year-old boy/girl,
c. 1958

8-year-old girl,
c. 1960

12-year-old girl,
c. 1951

12-year-old girl,
c. 1966

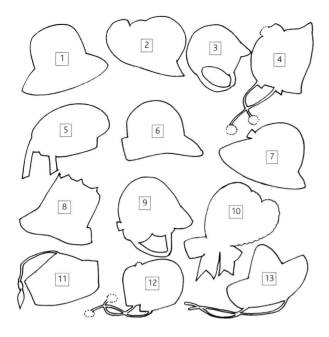

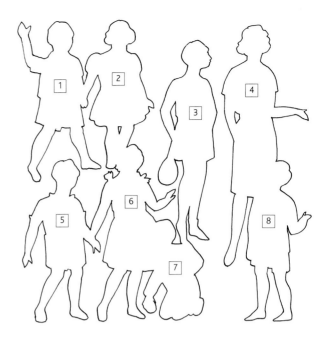

Hats 1934 – 1950

1 5-year-old girl, *c.* 1934. Felt hat with turned-down brim, wired edge trimmed with rows of top-stitching, matching seam at top of high crown and self-fabric bow on centre front, leather inner band. 2 5-year-old girl, *c.* 1935. Felt hat, heart-shaped brim turned up at front with multi rows of top-stitching, matching edges of seams on tall unlined crown, leather inner band. 3 6-year-old boy, *c.* 1936. Close-fitting leather fabric hat covering ears, small peak and narrow chinstrap with button fastening on one side, silk lining. 4 6-year-old girl, *c.* 1941. Close-fitting unlined knitted wool bonnet, pointed crown and double turned-back brim with contrast-colour wool pompon on centre front, matching ends of long rouleau ties. 5 8-year-old girl, *c.* 1950. Brimless checked wool beret with two-piece flat crown set onto narrow contrast-colour petersham ribbon band, matching bow with long ends in centre of crown. 6 4-year-old boy, *c.* 1937. Cotton hat, wide brim with multi rows of top-stitching, turned up at back and down at front, stitched detail repeated on edges of buttoned band and sections of tall crown. 7 6-year-old girl, *c.* 1938. Straw hat with wide wired brim narrowing at back, shallow domed crown with draped patterned silk ribbon band and matching bow on centre front. 8 12-year-old girl, *c.* 1940. Corded cotton hat lined with contrast-colour cotton, tall flat-topped crown cut into sections, seams on outside revealing lining fabric, detail seams continued through into deep brim, turned down at front and up at back. 9 4-year-old girl, *c.* 1944. Spotted cotton bonnet, close-fitting seamed crown, small peak and ear flaps with top-stitched detail, self-fabric chinstrap fastening at side with press stud under small bow. 10 8-year-old girl, *c.* 1947. Silk-covered hat with high crown gathered into self-fabric covered button on top, ruched heart-shaped brim, edges trimmed with contrast-colour ruched silk and bound with same, matching bow and ends at back, silk lining and satin inner band. 11 12-year-old girl, *c.* 1942. Chinese-style hat with deep padded satin-covered brim, flared out from head to partway up patterned silk-covered crown, pointed top with cord and tassel trim, silk lining, petersham inner band. 12 18-month-old girl, *c.* 1943. Close-fitting quilted silk bonnet trimmed on inner edge with a band of marabou feathers, matching pompon trim on ends of long rouleau ties, silk lining. 13 10-year-old girl, *c.* 1950. Holiday hat: natural straw with wide turned-back brim and tall pointed crown, long ribbon ties.

1934 – 1935

1 4-year-old boy, *c.* 1934. Striped cotton shirt, strap fastening with buttons in sets of three, tusks on either side from under yoke seam, Peter Pan collar, edges piped in contrast colour, matching cuffs on short sleeves. Plain cotton shorts with wide legs and top-stitched hems, worn with leather belt with round buckle. Short cotton socks with coloured trim. Leather shoes with T-straps, button fastenings, round toes and low heels. 2 5-year-old girl, *c.* 1935. Floral patterned cotton dress, fitted bodice with shaped inset band above knee-length gathered skirt with centre-front unpressed inverted box-pleat, plain cotton collar, matching cuffs on short puff sleeves. Bow-shaped plastic hair slide. Long knitted cotton socks. Leather shoes with bar straps, button fastenings and round toes. 3 8-year-old girl, *c.* 1934. Cotton tennis outfit: sleeveless bloused bodice with low V-shaped neckline edged with saddle-stitching, matching armholes, waist-belt and single breast pocket, above-knee-length divided flared skirt. Knitted cotton ankle socks. Canvas shoes with laced fastenings, round toes, rubber soles and low heels. 4 12-year-old girl, *c.* 1935. Printed check cotton dress, collarless bloused bodice with buttoned step fastening under high round neckline, edges decorated with top-stitching, matching hems of short sleeves, buttoned waist-belt and two hip-level patch pockets in knee-length straight skirt. Flesh-coloured stockings. Leather shoes with buttoned bar straps, round toes and low heels. 5 3-year-old boy, *c.* 1935. Pageboy outfit: velvet shorts with pointed waistline, buttoned to satin blouse with ruffled high round neckline, matching hems of short sleeves. Knitted cotton ankle socks. Patent leather shoes with buttoned bar straps, round toes and low heels. 6 5-year-old girl, *c.* 1935. Bridesmaid's outfit: sleeveless satin dress with bloused bodice, armholes bound with contrast-colour satin, matching high round neckline, bow trimming on each shoulder and wide velvet sash above knee-length full skirt. Knitted cotton ankle socks. Patent leather shoes with buttoned ankle straps, round toes and low heels. 7 3-year-old boy, *c.* 1934. Cotton blouse with Peter Pan collar above buttoned strap fastening and long sleeves gathered into buttoned cuffs. Contrast-colour cotton shorts with button-on braces. Heelless leather shoes with buttoned bar straps and round toes. 8 5-year-old boy, *c.* 1934. Hip-length knitted cotton shirt, pointed collar above buttoned strap fastening and long sleeves with sewn cuffs, short opening on side seams above hemline on either side. Corded cotton shorts. Knitted cotton socks with contrast-colour band at knee level. Leather shoes with buttoned T-straps, round toes and low heels.

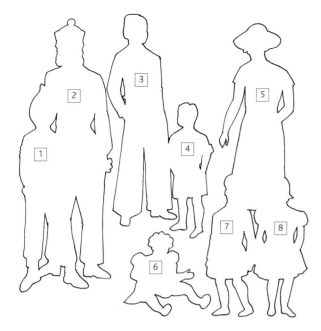

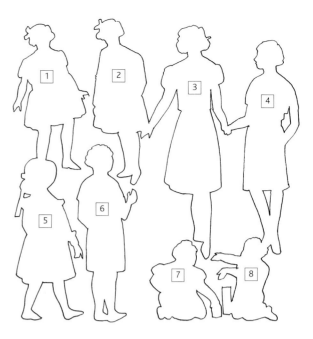

1936 – 1938

[1] 6-year-old girl, *c.* 1936. All-in-one padded waterproofed cotton ski suit: bloused bodice with diagonal welt pocket on either side of centre-front zip fastening, running from under high neckline with attached hood to crotch level, long raglan-style sleeves, wide self-fabric buckled waist-belt, long trousers gathered into knitted cuffs with large self-fabric patches from knee to ankle level, top-stitched edges and detail. Fur mittens with gauntlet cuffs. Leather ski boots with laced fastenings, round toecaps and low heels. [2] 12-year-old girl, *c.* 1937. Two-piece waterproofed cotton ski suit: hip-length jacket, bloused bodice with single chest-level patch pocket and asymmetric button fastening from under buttoned stand collar, matching waist-belt, cuffs on long shirt-style sleeves and ankle-level cuffs on full-length trousers, large self-fabric patches on front from knee to ankle, top-stitched edges and detail. Brimless knitted wool hat with soft crown trimmed with contrast-colour woollen pompon on top. Waterproofed cloth mittens. Leather ski boots with laced fastenings, round toecaps and low heels. [3] 9-year-old boy, *c.* 1937. Short checked wool jacket, semi-fitted body with diagonal jetted pocket on either side of centre-front zip fastening, wide collar and revers, adjustable side straps at waist level, long sleeves with buttoned strap above wrist level. Collar-attached cotton shirt worn with silk tie. Woollen trousers with hip-level pockets, fly fronts and wide legs with turn-ups. Leather shoes with laced fastenings, round toecaps and low heels. [4] 2-year-old boy, *c.* 1938. Cotton top, bloused bodice with double-breasted fastening, contrast-colour buttons, matching trim on sailor collar, cuffs on short sleeves, buckled belt and shorts. Long knitted cotton socks. Heelless leather T-strap shoes with button fastenings and round toes. [5] 12-year-old girl, *c.* 1937. Spotted cotton dress, fitted bodice with front button fastening, contrast-colour pin-tucked cotton asymmetric panel, matching corresponding panel in flared skirt, single hip-level pocket on opposite side skirt and back half of short sleeves, pointed collar, sewn cuffs on front half of sleeves and buckled waist-belt made on reverse side of spotted cotton. Straw hat, wide brim with wired edge and shallow crown. Flesh-coloured silk stockings. Leather shoes with buttoned bar straps and round toes. [6] 1-year-old girl, *c.* 1937. Sprigged cotton dress with high round neckline, short puff sleeves, full skirt and matching knickers. Short knitted cotton socks. Heelless cloth shoes with ribbon tie fastenings and round toes. [7] 4-year-old boy, *c.* 1938. Flecked wool tweed coat, asymmetric fastening with single velvet-covered button, matching button on narrow belt, Peter Pan collar, sewn cuffs on long sleeves and hip-level flap pockets in flared skirts. Flecked wool tweed peaked cap, sectioned crown with velvet-covered button trim on top, matching band. Knee-length knitted wool socks with wide turned-down cuffs decorated with contrast-colour bands. Leather shoes with laced fastenings, round toecaps and low heels. [8] 4-year-old girl, *c.* 1938. Cotton dress with fitted bodice, flared knee-length skirt, checked Peter Pan collar with plain contrast-colour cotton frilled edge, matching cuffs on short puff sleeves, edges of mock flap pockets set into piped waist seam and fabric of small round yoke. Straw hat with wide turned-down brim and tall domed crown with wide brightly coloured ribbon band. Short knitted cotton socks. Leather shoes with buttoned bar straps, round toes and low heels.

1939 – 1940

[1] 4-year-old girl, *c.* 1939. Knitted wool dress with fitted bodice above ribbed waistband, buttoned front fastening under patterned three-colour collar, matching short puff sleeves, tiny patch pockets and bands above hemline of full knee-length skirt. Ribbon bow worn in hair on one side. Short knitted cotton socks. Leather shoes with ankle straps, round toes and low heels. [2] 4-year-old girl, *c.* 1940. Double-breasted flecked wool tweed coat with semi-fitted bodice and flared skirts, velvet-trimmed collar, matching covered buttons and sewn cuffs. Ribbon bow worn in hair on one side. Short cloth gloves. Short knitted cotton socks. Leather shoes with T-straps, low heels and openwork decoration above round toes. [3] 12-year-old girl, *c.* 1939. Two-piece fine wool suit: waist-length collarless edge-to-edge jacket and matching knee-length flared skirt. Spotted cotton blouse with short puff sleeves, small collar and short necktie in matching fabric. Velvet ribbon bows worn in hair on either side. Short knitted cotton socks. Leather shoes with buttoned bar straps, round toes and low heels. [4] 9-year-old girl, *c.* 1939. Two-piece linen suit: short bolero-style collarless edge-to-edge jacket with short sleeves, single breast patch pocket and top-stitched edges and detail; flared knee-length skirt with centre-front inverted box-pleat, worn with buckled leather belt. Striped cotton blouse with single-breasted fastening and small collar. Short knitted cotton socks. Leather shoes with ankle straps, round toes and low heels. [5] 3-year-old girl, *c.* 1939. Unfitted patterned cotton coat, shoulder-wide collar with plain cotton frilled edge, matching trim above stitched cuffs on long sleeves, stitched tuck above hemline of full skirts. Natural straw hat with wide brim, high crown and ribbon band with bow at back and trailing ends. Short cotton gloves. Short knitted cotton socks. Leather shoes with ankle straps, round toes and low heels. [6] 3-year-old boy, *c.* 1940. Cotton satin shirt, small collar edged with lace, matching trim on hems of short sleeves. Knee-length striped wool trousers buttoned to blouse, on waistline front and back. Short knitted cotton socks. Leather shoes with T-straps, low heels and openwork design above round toes. [7] 2-year-old boy, *c.* 1940. Two-piece knitted wool suit: short top with contrast-colour ribbed collar, matching front buttoned strap fastening, yoke seam and cuffs of short puff sleeves; short trousers with elasticated waistband. Short knitted cotton socks. Heelless leather shoes with bar straps and round toes. [8] 2-year-old boy, *c.* 1940. Two-piece knitted wool suit: two-colour striped top with buttoned fastening on one shoulder to edge of collarless neckline, long sleeves with ribbed cuffs, matching hemline of top and hems of legs on short trousers. Short knitted cotton socks. Heelless leather shoes with bar straps and round toes.

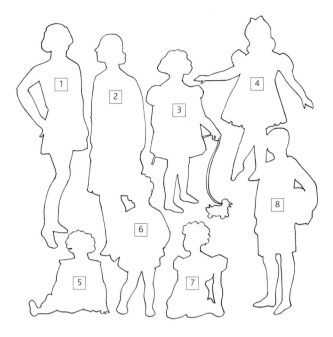

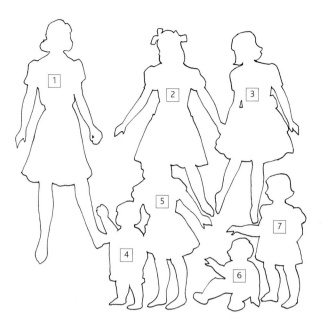

1941–1942

1 12-year-old girl, *c.* 1941. Two-piece striped cotton tennis outfit: bloused top with square neckline, bound in plain contrast-colour cotton, matching hems of short sleeves and tops of patch pockets on both top and on wide-legged shorts. Short knitted cotton socks. Lace-up canvas shoes with round toecaps, rubber soles and heels. 2 10-year-old girl, *c.* 1941. Fine wool sleeveless school dress with low square neckline, semi-fitted bodice and knee-length skirt cut in one piece, with box-pleats from under high yoke seam, wide self-fabric belt with back fastening. Plain cotton blouse with front button fastening under small collar and long sleeves gathered into buttoned cuffs. Cloth Alice band worn in hair. Lace-up canvas shoes with leather toecaps. 3 4-year-old girl, *c.* 1942. Short unfitted cotton dress with chest-level smocking from under rows of fine pin tucks, smocking repeated on short puff sleeves, plain contrast-colour collar above centre-front slashed opening with loop and button fastening, matching cuffs on short sleeves. Short knitted cotton socks. Leather shoes with buttoned bar straps, round toes and low heels. 4 4-year-old girl, *c.* 1942. Checked cotton gingham dress with high waistline emphasized by plain cotton inserted belt above short box-pleated skirt, matching narrow roll collar above double-breasted button detail and cuffs on short puff sleeves. Ribbon bow worn in hair at back. Short knitted cotton socks. Leather shoes with bar straps, round toes and low heels. 5 4-year-old girl, *c.* 1942. Spotted cotton dress with small plain cotton Peter Pan collar, matching covered buttons between collar and high yoke seam, short cap sleeves, above knee-length skirt with knife-pleats on either side. Short knitted cotton socks. Heelless leather shoes with bar straps and round toes. 6 3-year-old boy, *c.* 1941. Collarless single-breasted knitted wool cardigan with long sleeves. Cotton shirt with Peter Pan collar and concealed strap fastening. Short wool trousers buttoned to blouse front and back at waist level. Short knitted cotton socks. Leather shoes with bar straps and round toes. 7 4-year-old boy, *c.* 1942. Checked cotton two-piece playsuit: single-breasted blouse with plain cotton collar, matching covered buttons, mock handkerchief in breast patch pocket, cuffs on short puff sleeves and cuffs on short gathered knickers, deep waistband buttoned to blouse front and back. Short knitted cotton socks. Heelless leather shoes with bar straps and round toes. 8 7-year-old boy, *c.* 1941. Knitted wool tweed shirt with Peter Pan-style collar, buttoned strap fastening and long sleeves gathered into buttoned cuffs. Knee-length wool flannel shorts with side hip-level pockets, buttoned waistband, fly front fastening and centre-front creases. Knee-length knitted wool socks, turned-down cuffs with coloured band. Lace-up leather shoes with round toecaps and low heels.

1943–1944

1 12-year-old girl, *c.* 1943. Sleeveless lightweight wool pinafore dress, bloused bodice with sweetheart neckline, self-fabric inset waistband, knee-length bias-cut skirt with hip-level patch pockets, neckline and pockets with top-stitched detail. Patterned cotton blouse with frill-edged Peter Pan collar, matching edges of buttoned strap fastening, short puff sleeves with sewn cuffs. Short knitted cotton socks. Open-toe leather shoes with low stacked heels. 2 7-year-old girl, *c.* 1944. Knee-length patterned cotton dress with fitted bodice, gathered skirt, self-fabric belt set into side-front darts and fastening at back, plain cotton Peter Pan collar with frilled edge, matching turned-back cuffs on short puff sleeves. Hair ribbons worn on either side towards back. Short knitted cotton socks. Leather bar strap shoes with button fastening and round toes. 3 6-year-old girl, *c.* 1944. Cotton party dress with fitted bodice, short sleeves with self-fabric stitched cuffs, high round neckline with two decorative keyholes, edges bound with fancy braid, matching trim above narrow hip-level frill on gathered skirt, self-fabric belt set into side seams of bodice, tied into bow at back. Short knitted cotton socks. Heelless satin pumps with low-cut fronts, bow trim and round toes. 4 1-year-old boy, *c.* 1943. Cotton blouse with Peter Pan collar, buttoned strap fastening and short sleeves. Cotton shorts with wide braces buttoned at waist, wide legs with turn-ups. Knee-length knitted cotton socks. Heelless lace-up leather shoes with round toes. 5 4-year-old girl, *c.* 1944. Cotton dress with bloused bodice, narrow stand collar with contrast-colour pleated edge, matching sewn cuffs on short puff sleeves and tops of gathered hip-level patch pockets in full skirt. Three-quarter-length knitted cotton socks. Leather T-strap shoes with button fastenings, round toes and low heels. 6 Baby, *c.* 1943. Knitted wool romper suit, long sleeves with cotton cuffs, matching wide binding on high round neckline, top edge of patch pocket and wide band on hem of bodice, all-in-one combined legs and shoes buttoned to bodice on waistband. 7 3-year-old girl, *c.* 1944. A-line velvet dress with high round neckline edged with frill of lace, matching trim on narrow sewn cuffs on short puff sleeves and set into panel seams running from shoulders to flared hemline on either side of buttoned front fastening. Knee-length knitted cotton socks. Leather bar strap shoes with button fastening and round toes.

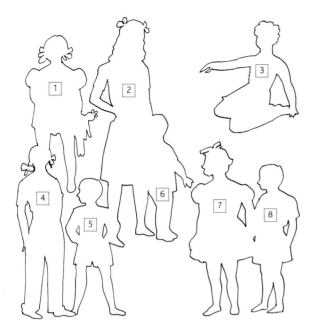

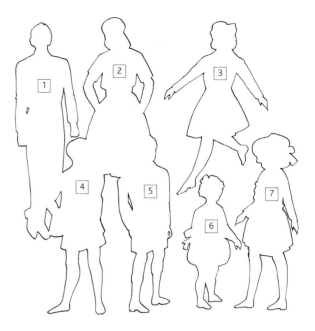

1945 – 1946

1 4-year-old girl, *c.* 1945. Cotton pinafore suit: sleeveless bodice with low square neckline, small patch pocket at hip level on one side of short culottes skirt and an embroidered rabbit on hemline of opposite side, top-stitched hems, edges and detail. Patterned cotton blouse with Peter Pan collar and short puff sleeves. Hair worn in bunches and tied with ribbon bows. Short knitted cotton socks. Leather shoes with buttoned bar straps and round toes.

2 12-year-old girl, *c.* 1946. Cotton shirt-style dress with bloused bodice, tucks on either side of front button fastening, shirt collar, high yoke seam, short sleeves with shoulder pads, wide self-fabric cummerbund, hip-level patch pockets in knee-length gathered skirt. Ribbon bows worn in hair on either side. Short knitted cotton socks. Sling-back leather sandals with T-straps and low heels.

3 3-year-old boy, *c.* 1946. Pageboy outfit: satin blouse with frill-edged Peter Pan collar, matching edge of front button fastening, short sleeves with sewn cuffs. Velvet shorts buttoned to blouse on high waist. Short knitted cotton socks. Leather shoes with buttoned bar straps and round toes.

4 6-year-old girl, *c.* 1945. Beachwear: hip-level patch pocket set onto one side of self-fabric frill-edged shorts, matching side seams and edge of bib top with wide shoulder straps. Heelless rubber beach shoes with buttoned bar straps and round toes.

5 7-year-old girl, *c.* 1946. Cotton denim trousers, wide legs with turn-ups, inset buttoned waistband, bib top with buttoned shoulder straps. Cotton blouse with shirt collar, front buttoned fastening, shoulder yoke seam, padded shoulders and short sleeves with sewn cuffs. Hair braids tied with ribbon bows. Canvas sandals with strap fronts, open toes and low heels.

6 5-year-old boy, *c.* 1945. Sailor suit: double-breasted top with full-length cuffed sleeves, single breast pocket and large collar trimmed with rows of braid, matching high round neckline of undershirt; shorts in matching fabric. Short knitted cotton socks with turned-down tops. Canvas lace-up shoes with low heels and round rubber toecaps.

7 5-year-old girl, *c.* 1945. Party wear: satin dress, fitted bodice with high square neckline outlined with bands of velvet, matching covered buttons of front fastening, binding on hems of puff sleeves, trim on hip-level patch pockets and band above hemline of full skirt. Ribbon bow worn in hair at back. Short knitted cotton socks. Leather shoes with buttoned bar straps, round toes and low heels.

8 4-year-old boy, *c.* 1946. Cotton shirt-style blouse, top-stitched collar, matching buttoned strap fastening, chest-level patch pocket and hems of short sleeves. Shorts in matching fabric, wide legs, front zip fastening and side hip pockets, worn with buckled leather belt. Knee-length knitted cotton socks. Lace-up leather shoes with round toecaps and low stacked heels.

1947 – 1948

1 12-year-old boy, *c.* 1947. Waist-length wool jacket with front zip fastening to under collar and revers, two chest-level patch pockets with zip fastenings, full-length cuffed sleeves with press-stud fasteners, waist-level buckled side adjusters. Cotton shirt worn with wool necktie. Straight-cut trousers with turn-ups and fly front. Slip-on leather shoes with round toes and low stacked heels.

2 10-year-old girl, *c.* 1948. Cotton dress, bloused bodice with decorative seams, self-fabric waist-belt tied at front, knee-length gathered skirt, low square neckline in-filled with contrast-colour cotton mock blouse with button fastening and shirt-style collar, matching sewn cuffs on short sleeves and inset detail on hip-level patch pockets. Stretch fabric hair band.

3 8-year-old girl, *c.* 1947. Double-breasted wool coat cut in flared panels without a waist seam, velvet-trimmed Peter Pan collar, matching covered buttons and hip-level shaped welt pockets in flared skirts. Hat in fabric to match coat, pointed crown, turned-back brim trimmed with velvet. Short knitted wool gloves. Short knitted cotton socks. Lace-up leather shoes with round toes and low heels.

4 6-year-old boy, *c.* 1947. Single-breasted collarless wool jacket with patch pockets. Knitted multicoloured striped wool jumper with high round neckline. Cotton shirt with large pointed collar worn with wool necktie. Wool shorts with fly front, hip-level jetted pockets and central creases. Knee-length knitted ribbed wool socks. Lace-up leather shoes with round toes and combined rubber soles and heels.

5 6-year-old boy, *c.* 1948. Two-piece wool suit: double-breasted jacket with wide revers, long sleeves and flap pockets; shorts with centre creases. Cotton shirt with long sleeves and pointed collar, worn with striped wool tie. Knee-length knitted wool socks with turned-down tops. Lace-up leather shoes with round toecaps and low stacked heels.

6 3-year-old girl, *c.* 1947. Bathing costume: bib with V-shaped neckline and front panel of gathered knickers, with side pockets, cut in one piece without waist seam, self-fabric waistband ties at back, multicoloured embroidered flowers under neckline and pockets. Small ribbon bow worn in hair on one side. Ankle-length knitted cotton socks. Leather sandals, T-straps with buckle fastenings, low heels and openwork above round toes.

7 5-year-old girl, *c.* 1948. Single-breasted wool coat with fitted bodice, small collar, full-length sleeves with sewn cuffs, half-belt at back with self-fabric covered button trim, knee-length pleated skirts. Natural straw hat with silk ribbon band and bow trim at back. Short cloth gloves. Short knitted cotton socks. Leather shoes, T-straps with buckle fastenings, round toes and low heels.

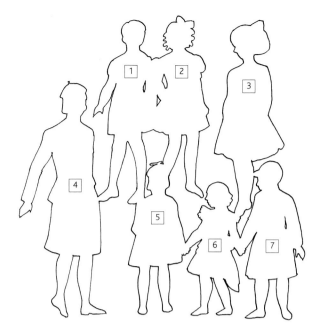

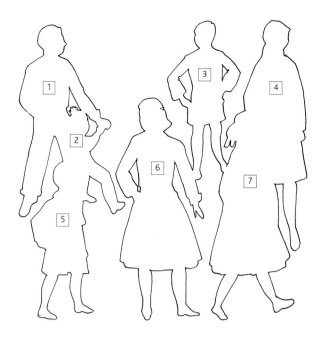

1949–1951

1 5-year-old boy, c. 1949. Checked cotton blouse with shirt-style collar, centre-front buttoned strap fastening and short puff sleeves with sewn cuffs. Wool shorts with buttoned waistband and wide legs with centre creases. Short knitted cotton socks. Lace-up leather shoes with round toecaps and low stacked heels. 2 5-year-old girl, c. 1950. Rayon dress with bloused bodice between inset smocked bands at chest and waist levels, high round neckline with frilled edge, matching hems of sewn cuffs on short puff sleeves, gathered skirt. Large ribbon bow worn in hair on one side. Short knitted cotton socks. Leather sandals with T-straps, low heels and openwork above round toes. 3 6-year-old girl, c. 1950. Beachwear: cotton sundress with ruched bodice topped with two rows of frills, wide shoulder straps, knee-length gathered skirt. Large natural straw hat with tall pointed crown and wide turned-back brim, ribbon ties under chin fastening on one side. Rubber beach shoes, bar straps with button fastenings, contrast-colour rubber soles and low heels. 4 12-year-old girl, c. 1951. Two-piece wool suit: single-breasted hip-length jacket with high rounded revers, collar trimmed with contrast-colour velvet, matching four flap pockets, long sleeves, padded shoulders; knee-length skirt with box-pleated front panel. Cotton blouse with button fastening, shirt collar and long sleeves. Wool beret with centre stalk. Short leather gloves. Short knitted cotton socks. Lace-up leather shoes with round toes and low heels. 5 4-year-old girl, c. 1951. Double-breasted wool coat, Peter Pan-style collar trimmed with velvet, matching covered buttons and edges of hip-level welt pockets, flared skirts, coat cut in one piece without waist seam. Beret-style hat with bow trim on top, matching coat fabric and trim. Short knitted wool gloves. Short knitted cotton socks. Leather shoes, bar straps with button fastenings, round toes. 6 3-year-old girl, c. 1950. Party wear: sleeveless artificial silk dress with wide neckline edged with two rows of frills and contrast-colour binding and bow, matching hip-level patch pockets in full skirt and colour of half-sash tied at back. Knee-length knitted cotton socks. Satin shoes with buttoned bar straps, leather soles and low heels. 7 5-year-old boy, c. 1951. School uniform: knee-length double-breasted wool coat with wide collar and revers, full-length raglan sleeves, wide self-fabric buckled belt and hip-level sloping welt pockets. Cotton shirt worn with plain wool tie. Wool cap cut into sections, school crest on front, wide stiffened peak. Short leather gloves. Long knitted wool socks with turned-down tops. Lace-up leather shoes with round toecaps and low stacked heels.

1952–1953

1 9-year-old girl, c. 1953. Winter sportswear: two-piece wool trouser suit consisting of waist-length top with bloused bodice from above wide waistband, low square neckline in-filled with self-fabric pleated scarf-effect, long cuffed sleeves and narrow trousers with turn-ups and centre creases. Hat in fabric to match suit with sectioned crown and turned-back peak, hat worn over bonnet with ties under chin. Wool mittens with flared cuffs. Lace-up leather shoes with round toes and low heels. 2 3-year-old boy, c. 1953. Winter sportswear: hand-knitted wool sweater with polo neck and long cuffed sleeves. Wool trousers with stirrups under feet. Hand-knitted two-colour wool hat with bobble trim. Leather shoes with round toes and low heels. 3 6-year-old boy, c. 1952. Waist-length wool jacket with front zip fastening under shirt-style collar, long sleeves gathered into cuffs and single chest-level patch pocket. Wool shorts with wide legs and centre creases. Three-quarter-length knitted cotton socks. Leather sandals with buckled T-straps, round toes and low heels. 4 10-year-old boy, c. 1953. Knee-length wool tweed overcoat with concealed fly front fastening under narrow collar and revers, full-length raglan sleeves and hip-level flap pockets, top-stitched edges and detail. Wool neck scarf, cotton shirt and wool necktie. Wool cap with crown cut in sections and narrow stiffened peak. Knee-length knitted wool socks. Lace-up leather shoes with square toes. 5 5-year-old boy, c. 1952. Hand-knitted wool sweater with cable design, high round neckline and long sleeves with turned-back cuffs. Wool shorts with turn-ups and centre creases. Knee-length knitted wool socks. Lace-up leather shoes with round toecaps and low stacked heels. 6 12-year-old girl, c. 1953. Striped wool dress with fitted bodice, narrow self-fabric buckled belt, button fastening under shirt-style collar and self-fabric tie, long sleeves with turned-back buttoned cuffs, hip-level welt pockets with button detail in knee-length flared skirt. Short knitted cotton socks. Leather slip-on shoes with high tongues, round toes and low heels. 7 8-year-old girl, c. 1953. School uniform: knee-length double-breasted wool coat with wide collar and revers, long raglan sleeves, hip-level vertical welt pockets set into side-front panel seams, hand top-stitched edges, seams and detail. Cotton shirt and wool necktie. Felt hat with turned-back brim, high crown with ribbon band and ends. Short leather gloves. Knee-length knitted wool socks. Lace-up leather shoes with round toes and low stacked heels.

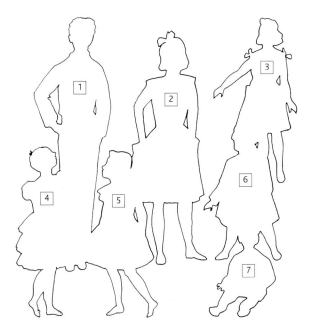

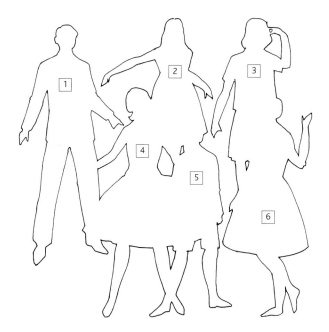

1954–1956

1 12-year-old boy, *c*. 1955. Machine-knitted wool collarless jacket with suede trim on either side of zip fastening, matching trim on side panel seams, long sleeves with buttoned cuffs, jacket bloused onto wide waistband. Knitted cotton shirt with pointed collar, cut to be worn open, long sleeves. Straight-cut wool trousers with fly front, side hip pockets and centre creases. Slip-on leather shoes with round toes. 2 10-year-old girl, *c*. 1954. Sleeveless spotted cotton dress with fitted bodice, waist emphasized by narrow buckled leather belt, square neckline and attached collar with ribbon braid trim, matching hip-level patch pockets in gathered knee-length skirt. Ribbon bow worn in hair on one side. Leather sandals with ankle straps, peep toes and combined platform soles and low heels. 3 7-year-old girl, *c*. 1954. Sleeveless patterned cotton dress, fitted bodice with square neckline edged with plain contrast-colour cotton, matching armhole bindings with bow trim on shoulders and trim on hip-length patch pockets in full skirt. Knitted cotton ankle socks. Leather shoes with crossed straps and round toes. 4 6-year-old girl, *c*. 1956. Party wear: cotton organdie dress, fitted bodice decorated with row of tiny buttons under tiny collar, short puff sleeves, knee-length three-tier gathered skirt trimmed with ribbon and edged with narrow self-fabric frills. Knitted cotton ankle socks. Patent leather shoes with buttoned ankle straps, low heels and bow trim above round toes. 5 6-year-old girl, *c*. 1956. Double-breasted shower-proofed cotton coat, fastening with buttons in two sets of four, small collar, long sleeves under gathered epaulettes, flared skirt and fitted bodice cut in one piece without waist seam. Shower-proofed cotton hat with sectioned crown and wide brim turned up at back. Short cloth gloves. Knee-length knitted cotton socks. Leather shoes with buttoned ankle straps, round toes and low heels. 6 3-year-old girl, *c*. 1955. Knee-length flared wool coat with off-centre button fastening under Peter Pan collar, long sleeves with split turned-back cuffs. Bonnet in matching coat fabric with sectioned crown and turned-back brim, strap under chin with button fastening on one side. Above-knee-length leggings in matching coat fabric, with side-button fastenings worn over heelless leather shoes with button fastenings and round toes. 7 1-year-old boy, *c*. 1955. Blouse with shaped yoke, contrast-colour Peter Pan collar, matching cuff on long sleeves, buttoned strap fastening and buttoned waistband on knickers. Short knitted cotton socks. Heelless cloth shoes with bar straps and round toes.

1957–1958

1 12-year-old boy, *c*. 1958. Single-breasted wool jacket fastening with brass buttons, wide collar and revers, long sleeves and three patch pockets, handkerchief in breast pocket. Cotton shirt worn with wool tie. Straight-cut trousers with turn-ups and centre creases. Lace-up leather shoes with square toecaps and low stacked heels. 2 6-year-old girl, *c*. 1958. Rayon dress with high waistline marked with large flat bow, sleeveless bodice with high round neckline, three outsized button fastenings and two chest-level welt pockets, knee-length flared skirt with box-pleats. Fabric hair band. 3 8-year-old girl, *c*. 1958. Knitted crimplene two-piece jumper suit: unfitted hip-length top with side panel seams, high round neckline faced in contrast colour, matching buttoned strap fastening, sewn cuffs on short sleeves and knee-length knife-pleated skirt. Knee-length knitted nylon socks. 4 12-year-old girl, *c*. 1957. Party wear: patterned man-made taffeta sleeveless dress with fitted bodice, low round neckline, contrast-colour band and bow set between side panel seams, matching detail above hemline on front panel and two horizontal bands in sides of full skirt, skirt worn over stiffened petticoats. Hair band. Nylon stockings. Leather pumps trimmed with tiny bow above pointed toes. 5 7-year-old boy, *c*. 1957. Two-piece wool flannel suit: single-breasted jacket with narrow collar and revers above three-button fastening, long sleeves trimmed at wrist with three buttons, two hip-level flap pockets; shorts with narrow legs and centre creases. Cotton shirt worn with wool tie. Knee-length knitted wool socks with turned-down tops. Lace-up leather shoes with round toecaps and low stacked heels. 6 10-year-old girl, *c*. 1957. Knee-length printed cotton dress, fitted bodice and bell-shaped skirt cut in panels without waist seam, mock belt-effect between panels at waist level, plain contrast-colour Peter Pan collar, matching turned-up cuffs on three-quarter-length sleeves, skirt worn over stiffened petticoats. Short knitted cotton socks. Leather shoes with decorative bar strap, pointed toes and low heels.

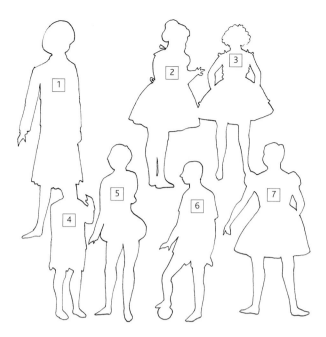

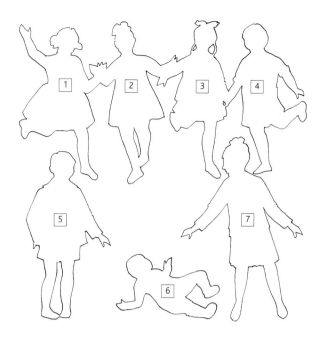

1959–1961

1 12-year-old girl, *c.* 1961. Two-piece wool suit: single-breasted hip-length jacket fastening with outsized self-fabric covered buttons, chest-level horizontal tuck with bow trim, pointed collar, full-length sleeves; knee-length knife-pleated skirt. Patterned silk blouse with pointed collar and long sleeves. Straw hat with wide turned-back brim. Short cloth gloves. Nylon stockings. Leather pumps with pointed toes and low heels. 2 6-year-old girl, *c.* 1960. Party wear: nylon velvet dress with fitted bodice, high round neckline, short puff sleeves and knee-length full gathered skirt, shoulder-wide nylon organza collar with velvet ribbon ties at back, matching trim on back waist. Long knitted nylon socks with turned-down tops. Patent leather shoes with decorative bar straps, pointed toes and low heels. 3 4-year-old girl, *c.* 1959. Holiday wear: sleeveless cotton sundress with bib front, wide shoulder straps with frilled edges, matching square neckline, hip-level patch pockets in full skirt and detail above hemline, multicoloured embroidery on shoulder straps, inset waistband and pockets. Short knitted cotton socks. Leather sandals with buckled bar straps, round toes and low heels. 4 4-year-old boy, *c.* 1959. Collarless single-breasted hand-knitted cardigan jacket fastening with leather buttons, cable pattern, long sleeves with turned-back cuffs. Knitted cotton shirt with pointed collar. Wool shorts with centre creases. Short knitted wool socks. Leather sandals with buckled T-straps, round toes and low heels. 5 5-year-old girl, *c.* 1959. Beachwear: cotton bathing costume, fitted bodice with self-fabric chest-level frill, low neckline with wide shoulder straps, attached knickers gathered onto bodice and gathered into band on hem. 6 5-year-old boy, *c.* 1960. Two-piece cotton playsuit: collarless single-breasted top with contrast binding on front edge, matching covered buttons, tops of two chest-level patch pockets, sewn cuffs of short sleeves and shorts with fly fronts and centre creases. Short knitted cotton socks. Leather sandals with buckled T-straps, round toes and low heels. 7 6-year-old girl, *c.* 1960. Party wear: cotton velvet dress with fitted bodice fastening at back with contrast-colour covered buttons, matching bow trim at base of fastening, frill-edged high round neckline, matching hems of sewn cuffs on short puff sleeves and hem of stiffened petticoat under knee-length full skirt. Knitted cotton tights. Patent leather shoes with buttoned bar straps, round toes and low heels.

1962–1963

1 4-year-old girl, *c.* 1962. Sleeveless cotton dress, fitted bodice with high round neckline and detachable contrast-fabric collar, full gathered skirt. Short knitted cotton socks. Leather sandals with buckled T-straps, round toes and low heels. 2 3-year-old girl, *c.* 1962. Sleeveless A-line wool flannel dress, high round neckline bound with self-fabric and trimmed on front with contrast-colour rouleau bow, repeated at base of centre-front channel seam and above inverted box-pleat. Knitted wool tights. Leather bar strap shoes with round toes and low heels. 3 4-year-old girl, *c.* 1963. Two-piece crimplene suit: single-breasted collarless jacket fastening with outsized buttons, hip-level flap pockets, long sleeves, hand-stitched edges and detail; box-pleated skirt. Ribbon bow worn in hair. Knee-length knitted nylon socks. Lace-up leather shoes with round toes and low heels. 4 4-year-old boy, *c.* 1962. Cotton blouse with Peter Pan collar, pin tucks on either side of buttoned strap fastening, short sleeves with turned-back cuffs. Wool shorts with shaped waistline and buttons onto blouse, wide legs with centre creases. Short knitted cotton socks. Lace-up leather shoes with round toecaps and low stacked heels. 5 5-year-old boy, *c.* 1962. Two-piece wool tweed suit: single-breasted jacket with three-button fastening, narrow collar and revers, two flap pockets, long sleeves with single button trim; shorts with fly front, wide legs with centre creases. Cotton shirt with pointed collar made to be worn open. Single-breasted hand-knitted wool waistcoat. Ankle-length knitted cotton socks. Leather sandals with buckled T-strap fastenings. 6 6-month-old baby, *c.* 1962. All-in-one machine-knitted romper suit with press-stud front fastening under tiny collar, long cuffed sleeves, combined legs and shoes. 7 8-year-old girl, *c.* 1963. Two-piece knitted wool jersey suit: unfitted hip-length single-breasted jacket, three-button fastening, Peter Pan collar, hip-level flap pockets and long sleeves; knee-length knife-pleated skirt. Short cloth gloves. Knee-length knitted cotton socks. Leather shoes with buttoned ankle straps and round toes.

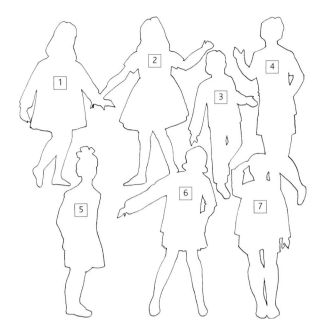

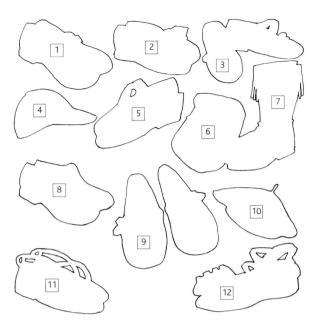

1964 – 1966

[1] 4-year-old girl, *c.* 1966. Cotton needlecord A-line dress, centre-front button fastening with plain contrast-colour velvet-covered buttons, matching ribbon bow under detachable shoulder-wide cotton collar, long sleeves with detachable cotton cuffs, hip-level patch pockets. Knee-length knitted cotton socks. Leather shoes with cross-over bar straps, round toes and low heels. [2] 5-year-old girl, *c.* 1966. Cotton dress, fitted bodice with deep scooped neckline in-filled with striped cotton, seam piped in self-fabric and trimmed with rouleau bow on centre front, piping repeated on hems of short sleeves and waist seam above gathered skirt. Wide ribbon Alice band worn in hair. Short knitted cotton socks. Leather shoes with buttoned ankle straps, round toes and low heels. [3] 3-year-old boy, *c.* 1964. Collarless single-breasted wool jacket with three-button fastening, long sleeves and hip-level patch pockets. Cotton shirt with pointed collar, worn with wool necktie. Wool flannel trousers with centre creases and without turn-ups. Lace-up leather shoes with round toes and low stacked heels. [4] 6-year-old boy, *c.* 1966. Machine-knitted multicolour striped cotton shirt with plain contrast-colour shirt collar and buttoned strap fastening, matching sewn cuffs on short sleeves and hip-level band on hem. Wool shorts with side hip pockets. Long knitted wool socks with contrast-colour patterned turned-down tops. Lace-up leather shoes with round toecaps and low stacked heels. [5] 4-year-old girl, *c.* 1965. Hip-length hand-knitted collarless and sleeveless cardigan tabard with multicoloured pattern, edged in plain colour, matching side-button straps, front fastening with hooks and bars. Machine-knitted cotton T-shirt with high round neckline and long sleeves. Knee-length cotton cord shorts, wide legs with turn-ups. Ribbon bows worn in hair. Knitted wool tights. Lace-up leather shoes with round toes and low stacked heels. [6] 6-year-old girl, *c.* 1965. Two-piece checked wool suit: hip-length collarless and sleeveless top, single-breasted fastening with leather-covered buttons, hip-level patch pockets; short knife-pleated skirt. Machine-knitted wool sweater with high polo neck and long cuffed sleeves. Hair held back with ribbons. Ribbed wool tights. Leather shoes with cross-over straps and round toes. [7] 6-year-old boy, *c.* 1966. Double-breasted wool tweed unfitted jacket with wide collar and revers, long sleeves, vertical hip-level welt pockets, hems, edges and detail edged with wool braid. Wool flannel shorts with centre creases. Hand-knitted sweater with high round neck and long sleeves. Knee-length knitted wool socks. Leather sandals with buckled T-straps and openwork detail above round toes.

Accessories 1951 – 1966

[1] 6-year-old boy, *c.* 1957. Leather shoes with buckled straps fastening over insteps, contrast-colour suede high tongues and front aprons, round toes, low stacked leather soles and heels. [2] 4-year-old boy/girl, *c.* 1951. Wool felt bedroom slippers with padded 'Noddy' heads on front, covering short tongues, top edges bound in contrast colour, round toes, combined rubber soles and heels. [3] 5-year-old girl, *c.* 1952. Coloured patent leather party shoes with buttoned bar straps, petersham ribbon bow trim above round toes, low stacked leather soles and heels. [4] 7-year-old boy, *c.* 1960. Fine wool school cap, close-fitting crown cut in sections with a contrast-colour inset band running horizontally through centre, button on top of crown, school emblem on front above stiffened peak. [5] 8-year-old girl, *c.* 1965. Leather shoes with double bar straps, linked on instep and buttoned on sides, round toes, low stacked soles and heels. [6] 5-year-old boy/girl, *c.* 1964. Hand-knitted three-colour patterned brimless wool hat with long pointed crown trimmed with large button and long tassel. [7] 12-year-old girl, *c.* 1959. Knee-length suede boots trimmed with leather binding and deep leather fringing around tops, matching inset piping around apron fronts, round toes, low stacked soles and heels. [8] 8-year-old girl, *c.* 1966. Textured leather shoes, laced through three eyelets above high tongues, hand-stitched edges and detail, round toes, low stacked soles and heels. [9] 6-year-old boy/girl, *c.* 1958. Leather sandals with buckled T-straps and fancy openwork on fronts above round toes, crepe soles. [10] 8-year-old girl, *c.* 1960. Imitation fur fabric beret set onto narrow band, stiffened stalk in centre of crown. [11] 12-year-old girl, *c.* 1951. Coloured patent leather shoes with low sweetheart-shaped vamps, cross-over ankle straps threaded through single loop at back of heel tops, side metal buckle fastening, round toes, low heels. [12] 12-year-old girl, *c.* 1966. Leather sandals with open strap fronts and peep toes, open sides, sling-back straps and ankle straps fastening with metal buckles, combined low wedge platform soles and heels covered in matching leather.

Accessories 1967–1982

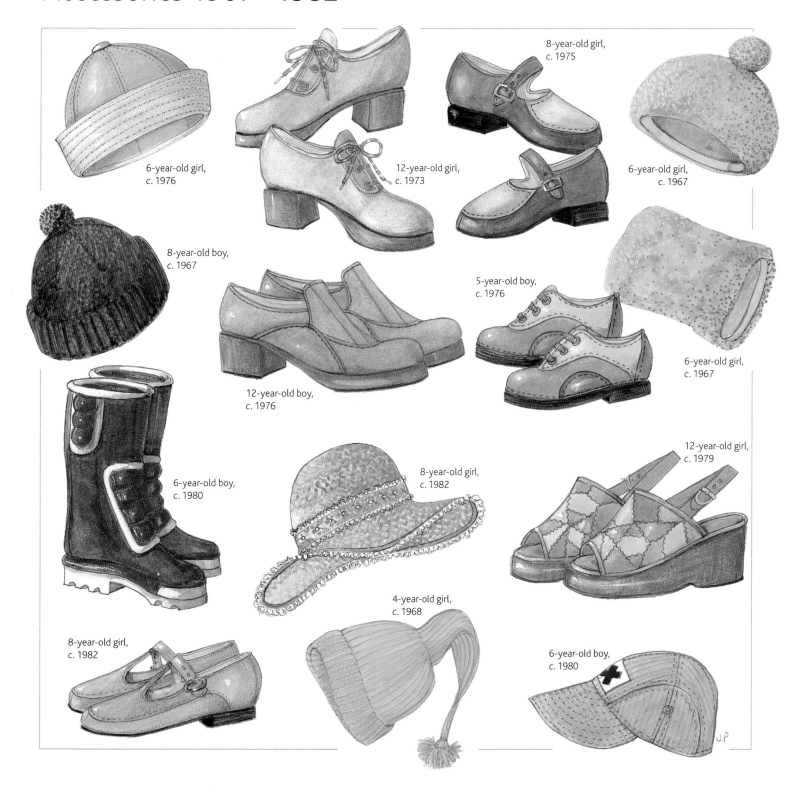

6-year-old girl,
c. 1976

12-year-old girl,
c. 1973

8-year-old girl,
c. 1975

6-year-old girl,
c. 1967

8-year-old boy,
c. 1967

5-year-old boy,
c. 1976

6-year-old girl,
c. 1967

12-year-old boy,
c. 1976

6-year-old boy,
c. 1980

8-year-old girl,
c. 1982

12-year-old girl,
c. 1979

8-year-old girl,
c. 1982

4-year-old girl,
c. 1968

6-year-old boy,
c. 1980

1967–1969

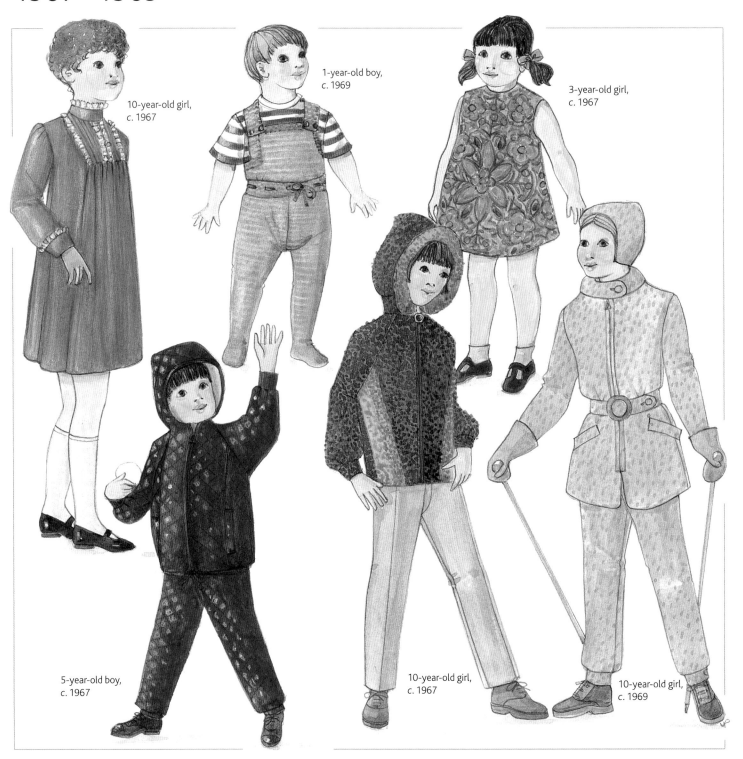

10-year-old girl,
c. 1967

1-year-old boy,
c. 1969

3-year-old girl,
c. 1967

5-year-old boy,
c. 1967

10-year-old girl,
c. 1967

10-year-old girl,
c. 1969

1970–1973

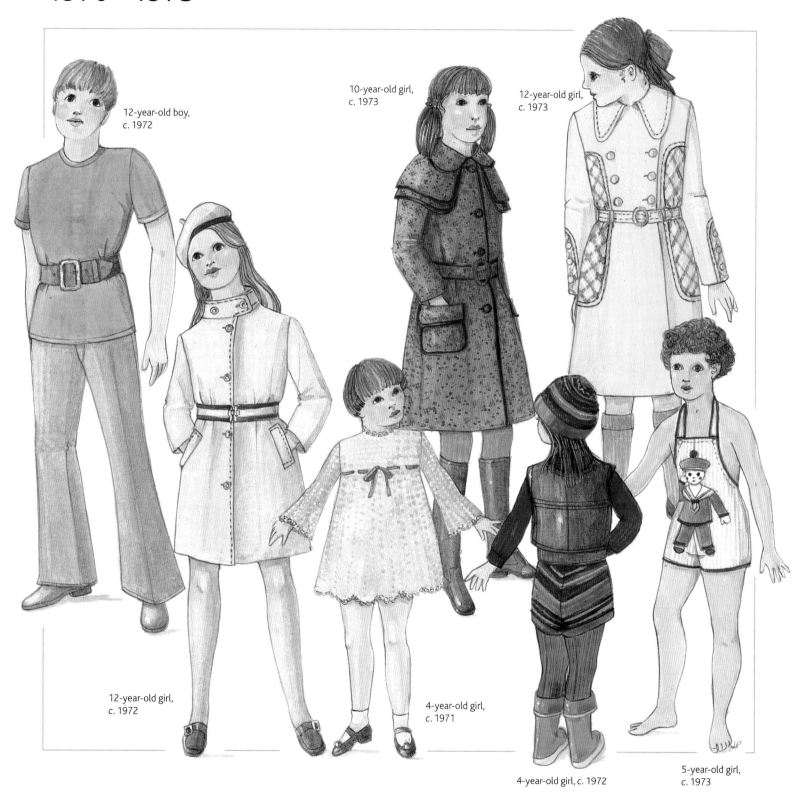

12-year-old boy,
c. 1972

10-year-old girl,
c. 1973

12-year-old girl,
c. 1973

12-year-old girl,
c. 1972

4-year-old girl,
c. 1971

4-year-old girl, *c.* 1972

5-year-old girl,
c. 1973

1974—1975

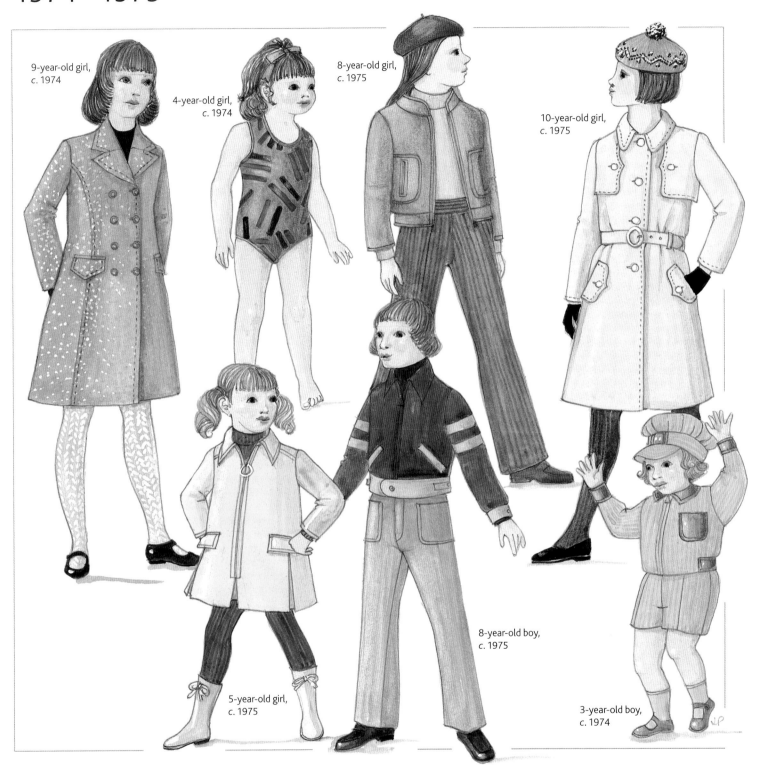

9-year-old girl, *c*. 1974

4-year-old girl, *c*. 1974

8-year-old girl, *c*. 1975

10-year-old girl, *c*. 1975

5-year-old girl, *c*. 1975

8-year-old boy, *c*. 1975

3-year-old boy, *c*. 1974

1976 –1977

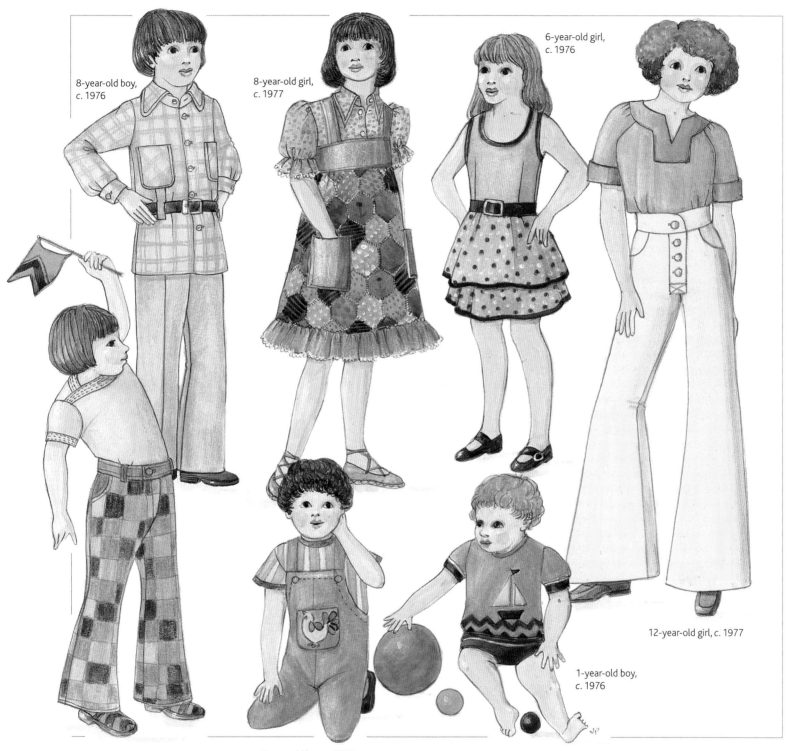

8-year-old boy,
c. 1976

8-year-old girl,
c. 1977

6-year-old girl,
c. 1976

12-year-old girl, c. 1977

1-year-old boy,
c. 1976

7-year-old boy, c. 1977

4-year-old boy, c. 1976

1978 – 1979

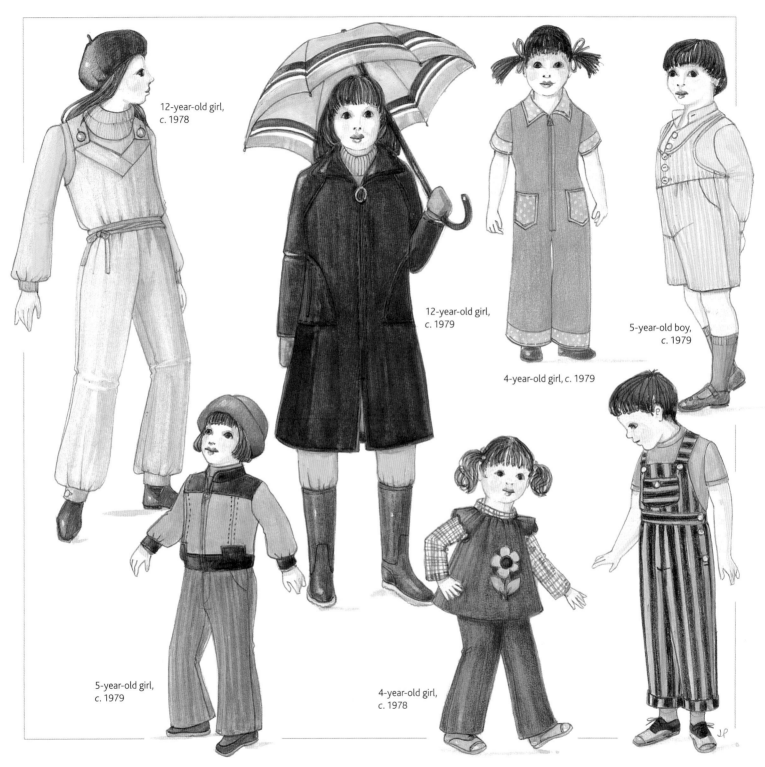

12-year-old girl,
c. 1978

12-year-old girl,
c. 1979

4-year-old girl, *c.* 1979

5-year-old boy,
c. 1979

5-year-old girl,
c. 1979

4-year-old girl,
c. 1978

6-year-old boy, *c.* 1979

1980–1981

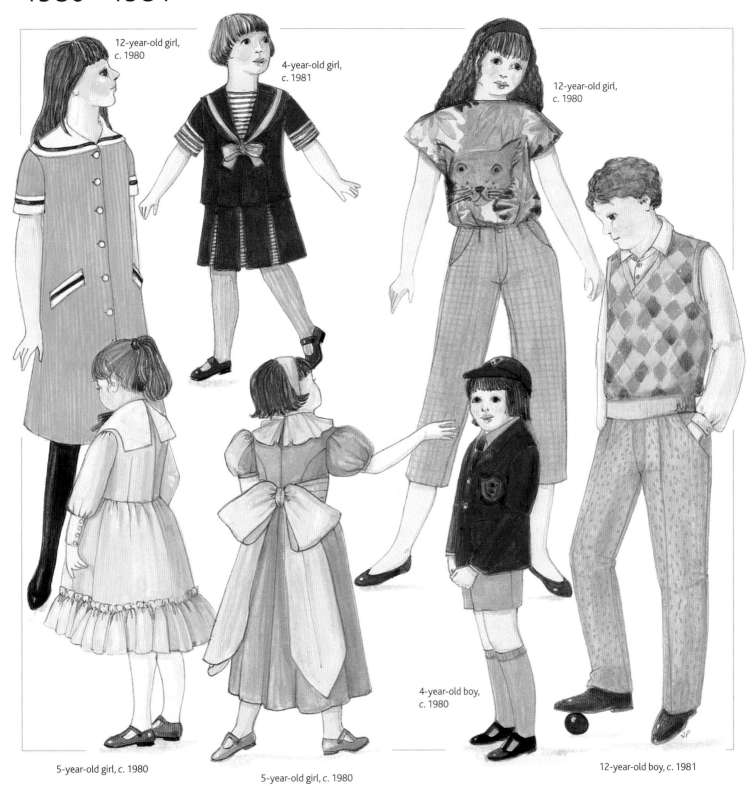

12-year-old girl, c. 1980

4-year-old girl, c. 1981

12-year-old girl, c. 1980

4-year-old boy, c. 1980

5-year-old girl, c. 1980

5-year-old girl, c. 1980

12-year-old boy, c. 1981

1982–1983

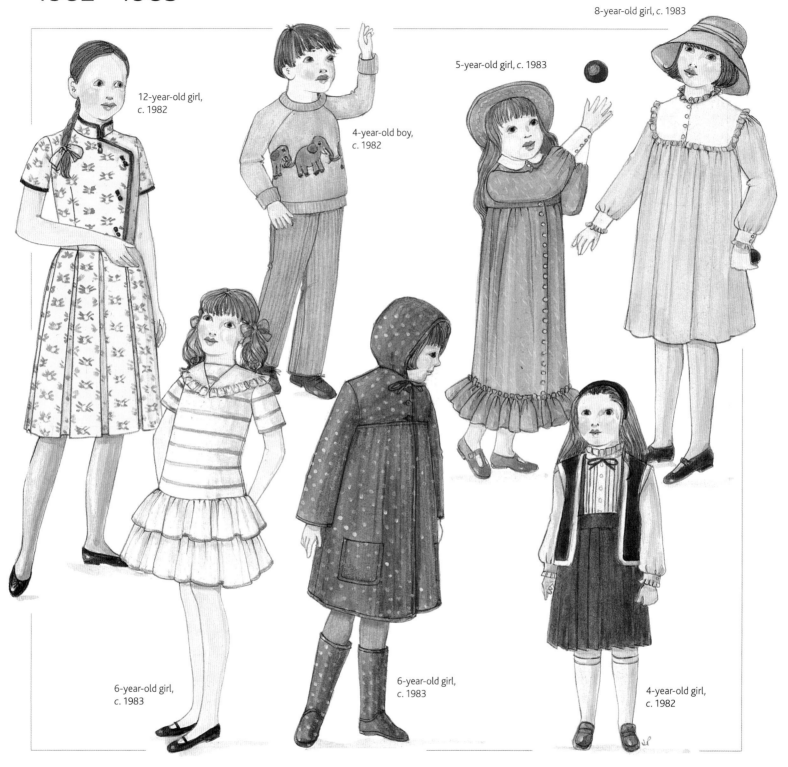

12-year-old girl,
c. 1982

4-year-old boy,
c. 1982

5-year-old girl, c. 1983

8-year-old girl, c. 1983

6-year-old girl,
c. 1983

6-year-old girl,
c. 1983

4-year-old girl,
c. 1982

1984–1986

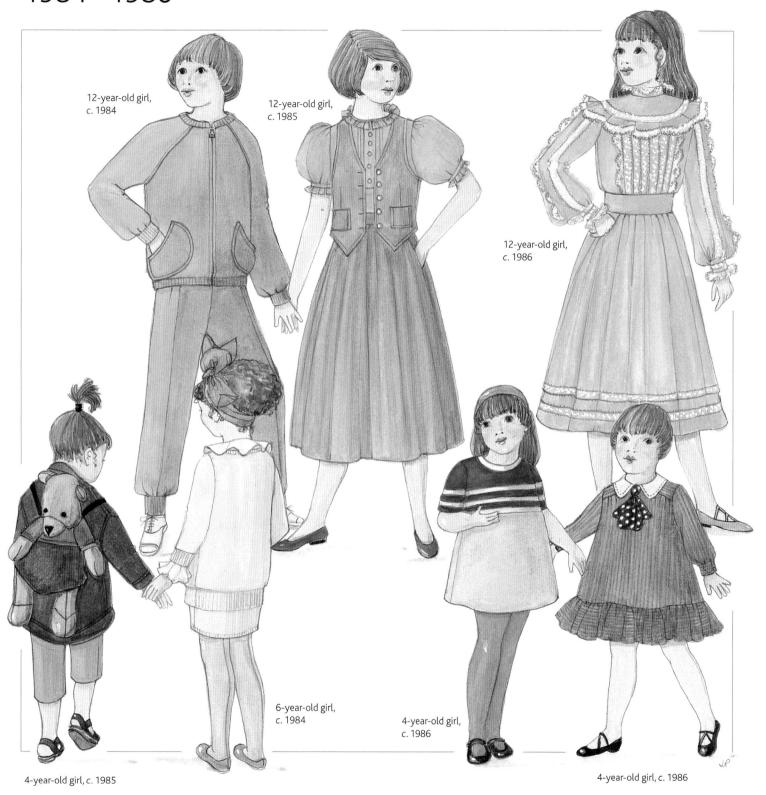

12-year-old girl, *c.* 1984

12-year-old girl, *c.* 1985

12-year-old girl, *c.* 1986

6-year-old girl, *c.* 1984

4-year-old girl, *c.* 1986

4-year-old girl, *c.* 1985

4-year-old girl, *c.* 1986

1987–1988

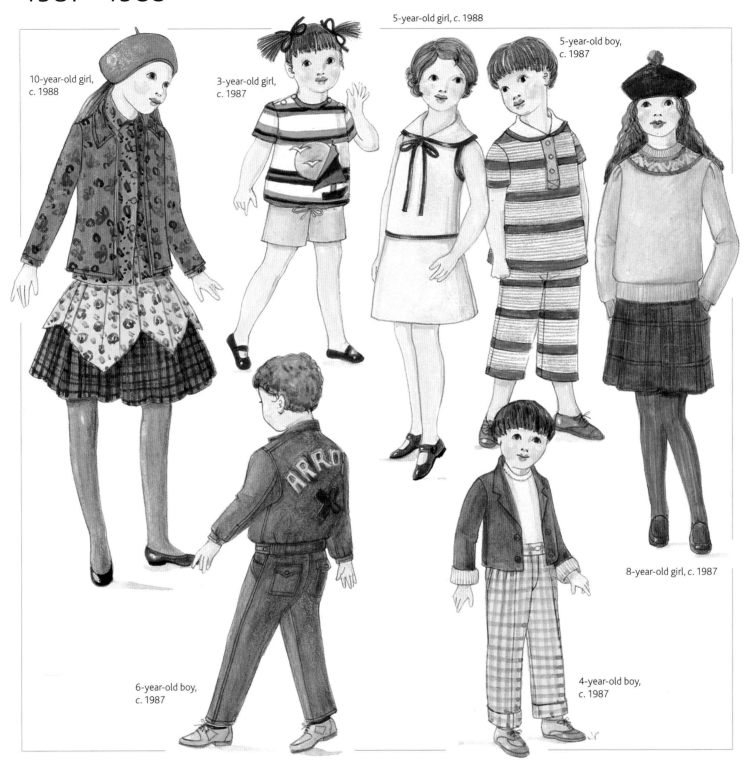

10-year-old girl, *c.* 1988

3-year-old girl, *c.* 1987

5-year-old girl, *c.* 1988

5-year-old boy, *c.* 1987

6-year-old boy, *c.* 1987

4-year-old boy, *c.* 1987

8-year-old girl, *c.* 1987

1989–1990

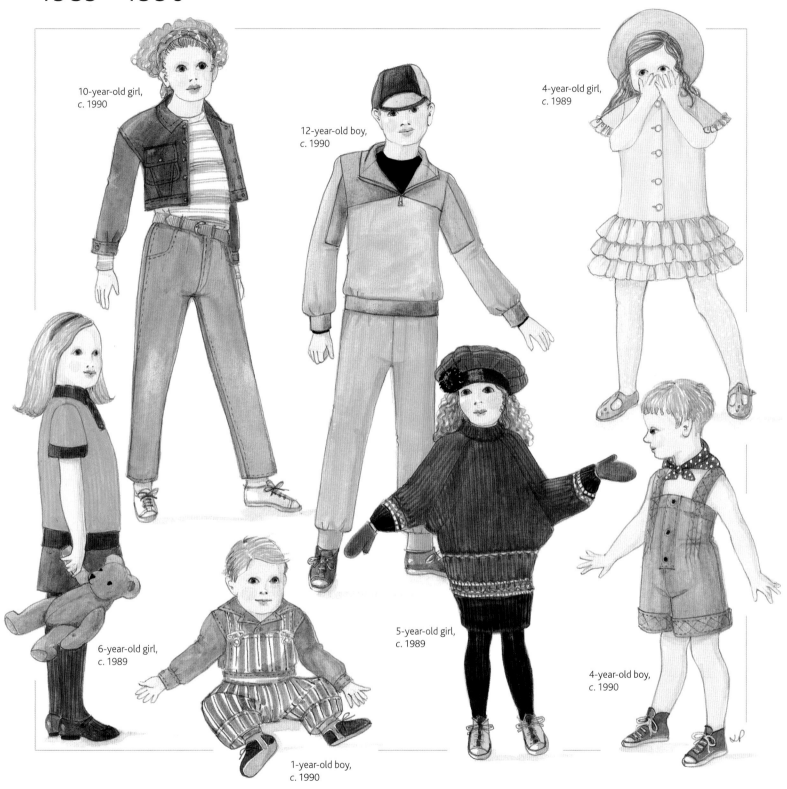

10-year-old girl,
c. 1990

12-year-old boy,
c. 1990

4-year-old girl,
c. 1989

6-year-old girl,
c. 1989

1-year-old boy,
c. 1990

5-year-old girl,
c. 1989

4-year-old boy,
c. 1990

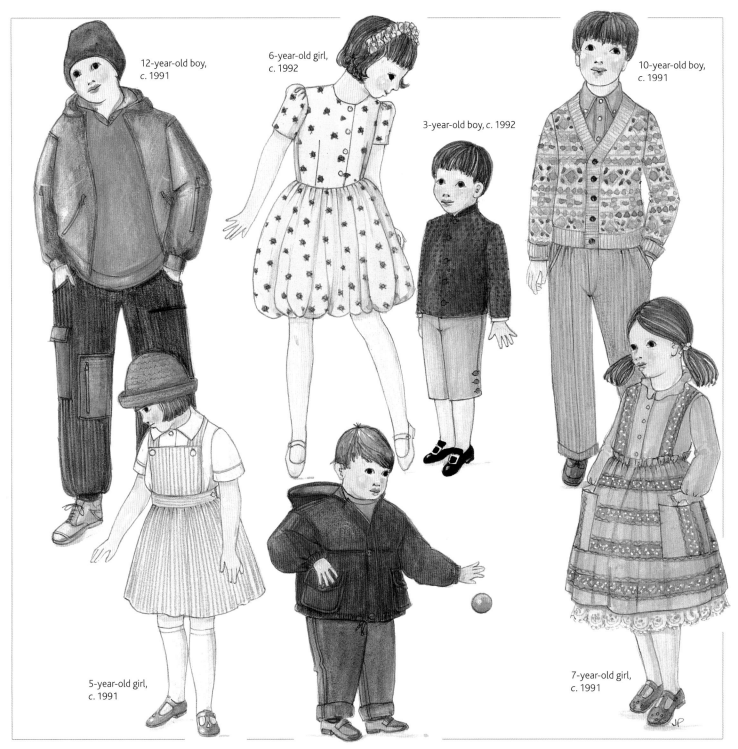

12-year-old boy,
c. 1991

6-year-old girl,
c. 1992

3-year-old boy, *c.* 1992

10-year-old boy,
c. 1991

5-year-old girl,
c. 1991

3-year-old boy, *c.* 1992

7-year-old girl,
c. 1991

1993–1995

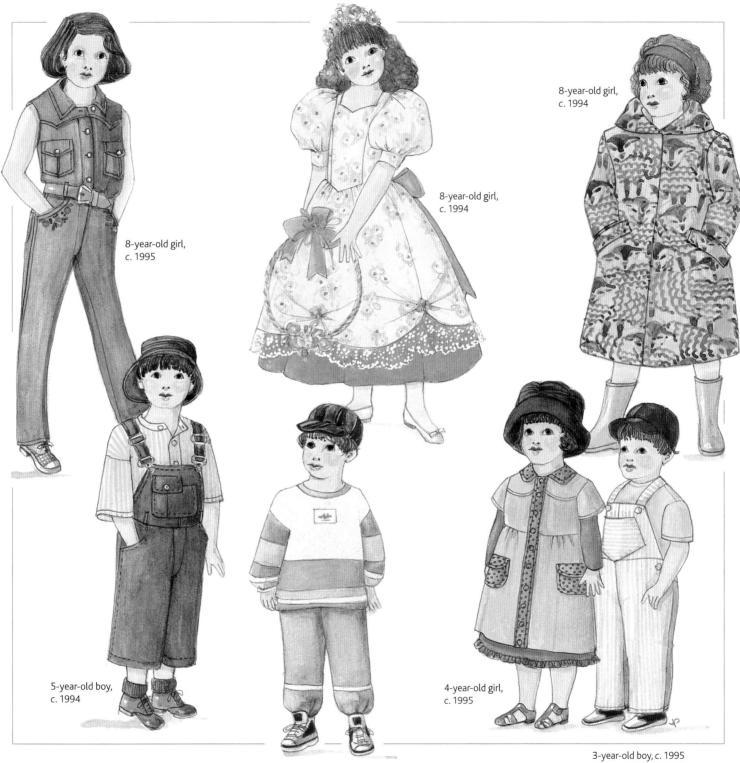

8-year-old girl, c. 1995

8-year-old girl, c. 1994

8-year-old girl, c. 1994

5-year-old boy, c. 1994

4-year-old boy, c. 1993

4-year-old girl, c. 1995

3-year-old boy, c. 1995

1996–1999

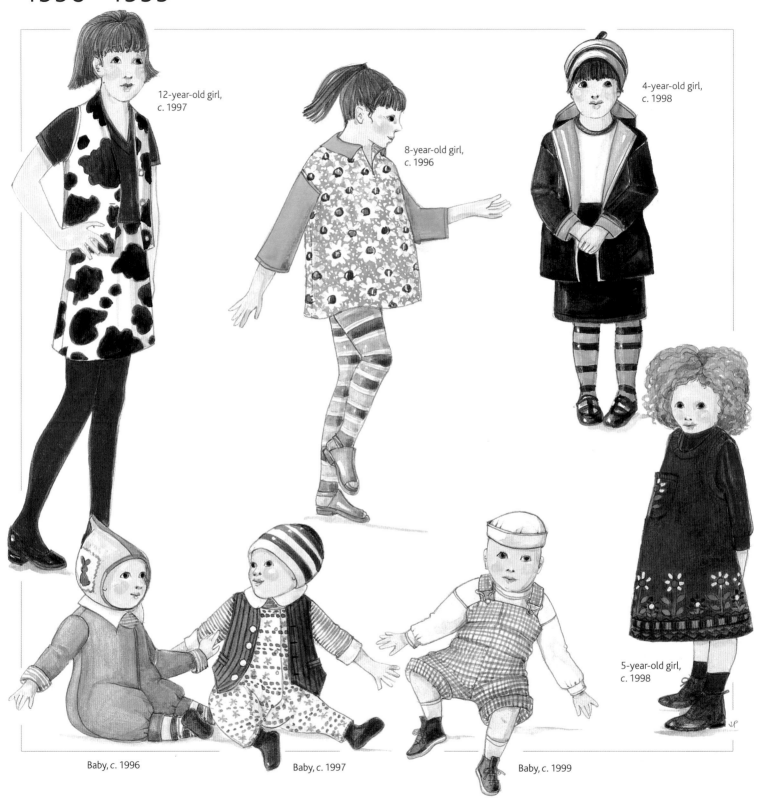

12-year-old girl,
c. 1997

8-year-old girl,
c. 1996

4-year-old girl,
c. 1998

5-year-old girl,
c. 1998

Baby, c. 1996

Baby, c. 1997

Baby, c. 1999

2000 – Present Day

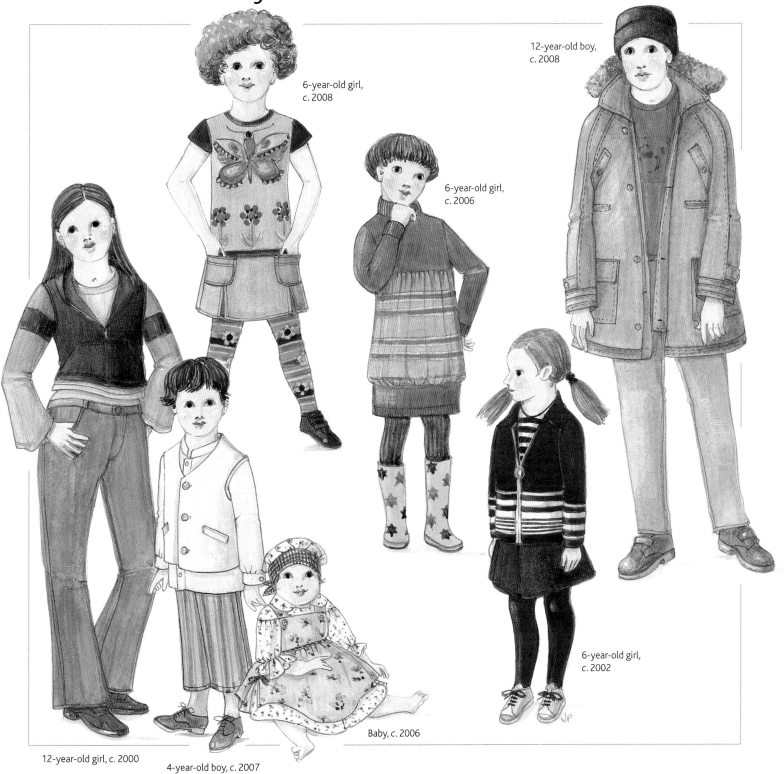

6-year-old girl,
c. 2008

12-year-old boy,
c. 2008

6-year-old girl,
c. 2006

6-year-old girl,
c. 2002

Baby, c. 2006

12-year-old girl, c. 2000

4-year-old boy, c. 2007

Hats 1983 – Present Day

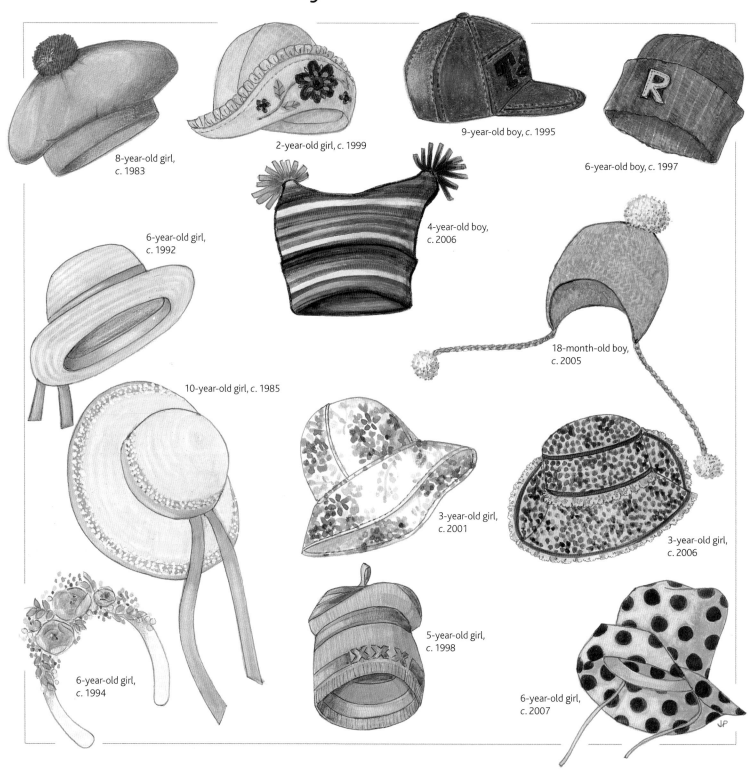

8-year-old girl, c. 1983

2-year-old girl, c. 1999

9-year-old boy, c. 1995

6-year-old boy, c. 1997

6-year-old girl, c. 1992

4-year-old boy, c. 2006

18-month-old boy, c. 2005

10-year-old girl, c. 1985

3-year-old girl, c. 2001

3-year-old girl, c. 2006

6-year-old girl, c. 1994

5-year-old girl, c. 1998

6-year-old girl, c. 2007

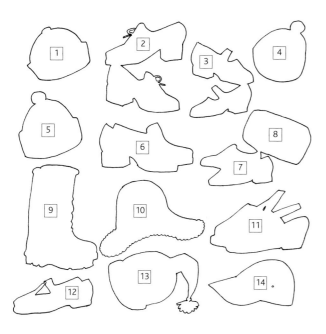

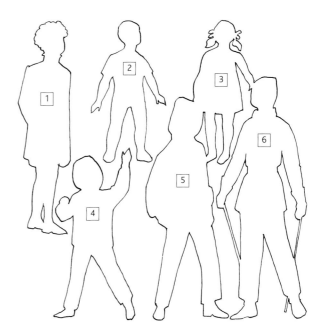

Accessories 1967 – 1982

1 6-year-old girl, *c.* 1976. Stiffened cotton satin hat with domed crown cut in sections, contrast-colour turned-back brim, matching covered button on top of crown, top-stitched brim, edges and detail, lined in unstiffened self fabric. 2 12-year-old girl, *c.* 1973. Lace-up leather shoes with high vamps and round toes, platform soles and thick heels covered in contrast-colour leather. 3 8-year-old girl, *c.* 1975. Leather shoes with buckled bar strap, apron fronts in pale-coloured suede with top-stitched detail, leather soles and low squat heels. 4 6-year-old girl, *c.* 1967. Brimless faux fur beret with pompon trim on centre of domed crown, silk lining and petersham ribbon band. 5 8-year-old boy, *c.* 1967. Hand-knitted wool hat, domed crown made in sections with pompon trim on top, turned-back ribbed brim. 6 12-year-old boy, *c.* 1976. Slip-on leather shoes with semi-circular panels on either side of high tongues, round toes, platform soles and thick heels covered in contrast-colour leather. 7 5-year-old boy, *c.* 1976. Lace-up leather shoes with semi-circular panels on either side, matching colour of back heels, round toes, uppers and upper side panels in contrast-colour leather, upper parts with eyelets, in pale-coloured suede. 8 6-year-old girl, *c.* 1967. Faux fur hand muff lined with silk and edged, inside, with petersham ribbon band. 9 6-year-old boy, *c.* 1980. Mid-calf-length woven nylon boots with contrast-colour moulded soft plastic panels above round toes and on upper sides, under top edges, edges bound in second contrast colour, matching ribbed rubber platform soles and thick heels. 10 8-year-old girl, *c.* 1982. Natural straw hat with high domed crown, embroidered band edged with lace, matching edge of wide brim. 11 12-year-old girl, *c.* 1979. Patchwork leather shoes with open toes, sling-back straps with side-buckled fastenings, platform cork soles and medium-high wedge heels covered in contrast-colour leather. 12 8-year-old girl, *c.* 1982. Leather shoes with top-stitched apron fronts and T-straps with side-buckled fastenings, leather soles, round toes and low stacked heels. 13 4-year-old girl, *c.* 1968. Hand-knitted hat with elongated point ending in self-fabric pompon, turned-back ribbed brim. 14 6-year-old boy, *c.* 1980. Stiffened striped cotton cap with semi-circular panels above ears on sides, large peak with top-stitched detail, matching edges and detail.

1967 – 1969

1 10-year-old girl, *c.* 1967. Fine cotton mini-length shift dress with high waistline under lace-frill-trimmed yoke, matching edge of high stand collar and cuffs on full-length sleeves. Knee-length knitted cotton socks. Leather shoes with bar straps, round toes and low heels. 2 1-year-old boy, *c.* 1969. Hand-knitted playsuit with bib front, buttoned shoulder straps, inset drawstring waistband above full-length trousers with feet. Striped machine-knitted T-shirt with high round neckline and wide short sleeves. 3 3-year-old girl, *c.* 1967. Collarless and sleeveless mini-length A-line dress with outsized printed pattern of flowers and leaves. Hair worn in bunches tied with ribbon bows. Ankle-length knitted cotton socks. T-strap leather shoes with button fastenings, round toes and low heels. 4 5-year-old boy, *c.* 1967. Quilted and padded nylon winter playsuit: hooded top with front zip fastening, vertical welt pockets set into side panel seams, full-length raglan sleeves gathered into knitted cuffs; matching trousers. Lace-up leather boots with round toecaps and low heels. 5 10-year-old girl, *c.* 1967. Hip-length faux fur hooded ski jacket with front zip fastening, full-length sleeves gathered into cuffs, narrow inset side panels in two contrasting colours, matching edge of hood. Straight-cut full-length wool trousers with centre-front pin tucks and central fly fastening. 6 10-year-old girl, *c.* 1969. Two-piece wool tweed ski suit: hip-length jacket with centre-front zip fastening under wrap-over collar with button fastening, matching fastening to one side of buckled belt, hip-level welt pockets, full-length sleeves; straight-cut trousers gathered into buttoned band at ankle level. Wool tweed brimless bonnet to match suit. Leather gauntlet mittens. Leather ski boots.

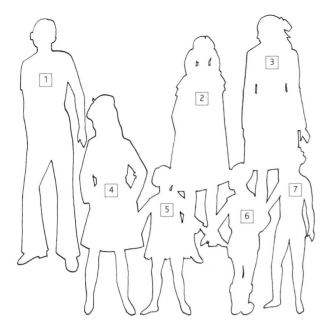

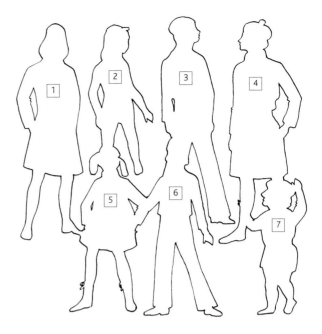

1970–1973

1 12-year-old boy, *c.* 1972. Knitted cotton T-shirt with high round neck and short sleeves, worn with wide leather waist-belt with large metal buckle. Cotton trousers with wide flared legs, central creases and fly front fastening. Leather shoes with platform soles, broad round toes and low stacked heels. 2 10-year-old girl, *c.* 1973. Single-breasted wool tweed coat with large collar, following lines of double shoulder cape, full-length sleeves, wide self-fabric waist-belt with large round plastic buckle, hip-level patch pockets with flaps, edges and detail bound with contrast colour. Hair worn in bunches secured with coloured elastic bands. Ribbed wool tights. Knee-length leather boots with round toes and low stacked heels. 3 12-year-old girl, *c.* 1973. Double-breasted wool coat with large collar, checked wool side panels set into fitted bodice and flared skirts, matching button-trimmed panels above wrist level on full-length sleeves. Large ribbon bow worn in hair at back. Knee-length knitted wool socks. Leather shoes with low heels. 4 12-year-old girl, *c.* 1972. Single-breasted wool gabardine coat with double-breasted stand collar, full-length sleeves, hip-level vertical welt pockets, contrast-colour saddle-stitched edges and detail, coat worn with elasticated waist-belt with centre-front clasp fastening. Brimless wool gabardine beret with stalk in centre of crown, contrast-colour petersham band. Knitted wool tights. Leather shoes with buckled straps above apron fronts and round toes. 5 4-year-old girl, *c.* 1971. A-line crocheted cotton mini-length dress with high round neckline, full-length flared sleeves with scalloped hemline, matching hem of skirt, high waist position marked by threaded velvet ribbon and bow. Knitted cotton ankle socks. Leather shoes with buttoned bar straps, low heels and rosette trim above round toes. 6 4-year-old girl, *c.* 1972. Short collarless and sleeveless leather waistcoat with top-stitched edges and seams. Hand-knitted wool sweater with polo neck and long cuffed sleeves. Hand-knitted multicolour wool striped shorts, matching pull-on hat with turned-back brim. Knitted wool ribbed tights. Mid-calf-length plastic boots with turned-down cuffs edged in contrast colour, matching edges of soles. 7 5-year-old girl, *c.* 1973. One-piece striped stretch cotton swimsuit, bib front with appliqué sailor, contrast-colour bound edges, matching rouleau shoulder straps and hems of shorts.

1974–1975

1 9-year-old girl, *c.* 1974. Double-breasted wool tweed coat with wide collar and revers, long sleeves, hip-level flap pockets, curved panel seams from chest level to hem of knee-length flared skirts, hand-stitched edges and detail. Plain knitted cotton T-shirt with high round neckline and long sleeves. Knitted wool tights. Coloured patent leather shoes with buttoned bar straps, round toes and low heels. 2 4-year-old girl, *c.* 1974. Multicoloured patterned stretch fabric swimsuit with low round neckline and cut-away armholes. Ribbon bow worn in hair. 3 8-year-old girl, *c.* 1975. Waist-length leather jacket with centre-front zip fastening from waistband to under stand collar, long sleeves, jetted pockets set inside leather patch. Knitted cotton T-shirt with high polo neck and long sleeves. Cotton cord trousers with wide waistband and flared legs. Wool beret with spike in centre of crown. Slip-on leather shoes with apron fronts, round toes and low stacked heels. 4 10-year-old girl, *c.* 1975. Single-breasted wool coat with large collar, long sleeves, mock bolero jacket with button detail, matching hip-level welt pockets, wide self-fabric belt with large round buckle. Hand-knitted two-colour patterned wool beret with pompon trim. Short leather gloves. Knitted wool tights. Leather pumps with low-cut vamps, round toes and low heels. 5 5-year-old girl, *c.* 1975. Plastic A-line dress with centre-front zip fastening from flared hem to under large pointed collar, high yoke seam, long sleeves and hip-level flap pockets. Knitted sweater with high polo neck and long sleeves. Knitted wool tights. Three-quarter-length plastic boots with rouleau bow trim on front, round toes, leather soles and low heels. 6 8-year-old boy, *c.* 1975. Waist-length leather jacket with centre-front zip fastening from waistband to under high collar, long sleeves with contrast-colour leather cuffs, matching two inset bands on upper sleeve, two diagonal welt pockets and wide waistband. Knitted cotton sweater with polo neck and long sleeves. Cotton trousers with flared legs, fly fronts and large hip-level patch pockets. Slip-on leather shoes with apron fronts, round toes and low stacked heels. 7 3-year-old boy, *c.* 1974. Two-piece striped cotton suit: waist-length top with centre-front zip fastening, small contrast-colour collar, matching cuffs on long sleeves, single breast pocket and half belt; shorts with centre creases. Cap with gathered crown and peak in matching fabric and trim. Short knitted cotton socks. Heelless coloured patent leather shoes with buttoned bar straps and round toes.

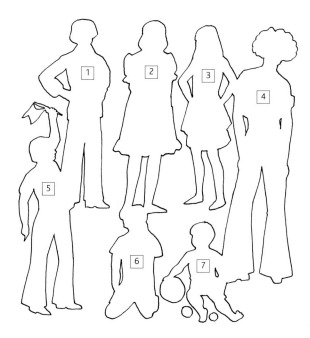

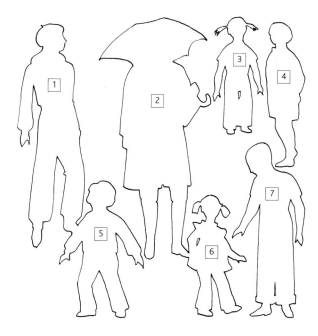

1976 –1977

1 8-year-old boy, *c.* 1976. Checked wool shirt with large collar, full-length sleeves gathered into cuffs, two large chest-level patch pockets, shirt worn with metal-buckled leather belt threaded though waist-level carriers. Flared wool trousers with central creases. Leather shoes with platform soles and stacked heels. 2 8-year-old girl, *c.* 1977. Patchwork printed cotton pinafore dress, plain cotton yoke bodice with shoulder straps, matching hip-level patch pockets and lace-edged hem frill. Spotted cotton blouse with large pointed collar and short puff sleeves with lace-edged frill. Canvas shoes with ribbon crossed straps and rope platform soles. 3 6-year-old girl, *c.* 1976. Knitted cotton dress, sleeveless fitted bodice with low neckline, edges bound in contrast colour, matching metal-buckled waist-belt and hems of two-tier patterned cotton skirt. Leather shoes with buckled bar straps, round toes and low heels. 4 12-year-old girl, *c.* 1977. Cotton blouse, high round neckline with centre-front nick, edged with contrast-colour cotton, matching cuffs on short raglan-style sleeves. Stiff cotton trousers with wide flared legs, deep waistband, hip-level pockets and front fastening with self-fabric covered buttons. Leather shoes with apron fronts, round toes and low heels. 5 7-year-old boy, *c.* 1977. Knitted cotton T-shirt with top-stitched cross-over neckline, matching hems of short sleeves. Patchwork denim trousers with wide waistband, side pockets, fly fronts and flared legs. Knitted cotton socks. Plastic sandals with thick soles and low heels. 6 4-year-old boy, *c.* 1976. Cotton overalls, bib front with buttoned straps, appliqué bird on single patch pocket, legs with feet. Striped knitted cotton T-shirt with high round neckline edged in contrast colour, matching hems of short sleeves. Heelless cloth slippers with round toes. 7 1-year-old boy, *c.* 1976. Cotton shirt with high round neckline and short sleeves with contrast-colour cuffs, matching bound hemline under colourful print of sailing ship and sea.

1978 –1979

1 12-year-old girl, *c.* 1978. Wool flannel overalls, sleeveless bloused bodice with low V-shaped neckline and wide shoulder straps with large self-fabric covered button fastenings, self-fabric rouleau belt wound twice around waist and tied into bow on one side, straight-cut trousers gathered into buttoned cuffs at ankle level. Wool beret with central stalk. Elastic-sided leather ankle boots with square toes and low heels. 2 12-year-old girl, *c.* 1979. Knee-length plastic raincoat with centre-front zip fastening from under wing collar, full-length raglan sleeves, waist-level curved triangular patch pockets with vertical jetted openings, top-stitched edges and detail. Polo neck sweater. Leather mittens. Multicolour striped umbrella with thick handle. Trousers tucked into knee-length leather boots with round toes and combined crepe soles and heels. 3 4-year-old girl, *c.* 1979. One-piece cotton playsuit with centre-front zip fastening from under spotted cotton collar, matching cuffs on short sleeves, hip-level patch pockets and cuffs on hems of wide legs. Hair worn in bunches and tied with ribbon bows. Heelless leather shoes with round toes. 4 5-year-old boy, *c.* 1979. One-piece striped cotton playsuit, sleeveless single-breasted waistcoat-style bodice with low neckline, above-knee-length trousers with hip-level pockets. Collarless cotton shirt with long sleeves gathered into cuffs. Knee-length knitted cotton socks. Leather sandals with buckled bar straps, openwork detail above round toes, leather soles and low heels. 5 5-year-old girl, *c.* 1979. Waist-length leather jacket with suede yoke, matching stand collar, waist-level band with inset pockets and cuffs on long sleeves, top-stitched seams on either side of centre-front zip fastening. Knitted cotton polo neck sweater with long sleeves. Cotton velvet needlecord flared trousers with hip-level pockets and fly front. Pull-on wool hat with padded turned-back brim. Leather shoes with apron fronts, combined crepe soles and heels. 6 4-year-old girl, *c.* 1978. Two-piece cotton playsuit: hip-level flared top gathered from under checked cotton stand collar, matching long sleeves from under self-fabric cap sleeves, large appliqué flower motif on front; straight-cut trousers in matching fabric. Hair worn in bunches and secured with elastic bands. Lace-up canvas trainers with rubber toecaps and combined soles and heels. 7 6-year-old boy, *c.* 1979. Striped cotton overalls, bib front with single patch pocket with button trim and buttoned straps, inset waistband buttoned on one side above buttoned opening in side seam of ankle-length trousers with wide turn-ups. Knitted cotton T-shirt with high round neckline and short sleeves. Striped knitted cotton socks. Multicoloured trainers with combined rubber soles and heels.

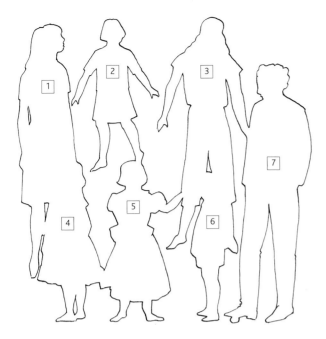

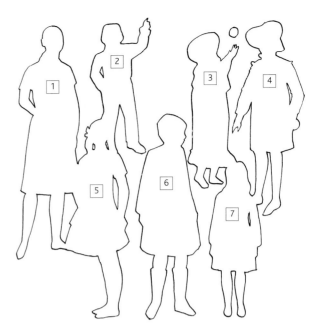

1980 –1981

1 12-year-old girl, *c*. 1980. Striped cotton needlecord knee-length shift dress with single-breasted button fastening, shoulder-wide plain cotton collar with contrast-colour ribbon border, matching cuffs on short sleeves and hip-level welt pockets. Wool tights. Leather shoes with pointed toes. 2 4-year-old girl, *c*. 1981. Two-piece wool jersey suit: hip-level panelled top with wide sailor collar banded with ribbon and trimmed with a centre-front bow, ribbon detail repeated above striped bands on short sleeves, striped vest under low neckline, matching inside of box-pleats in knee-length skirt. Ribbed wool tights. Leather shoes with buttoned bar straps, contrast-colour soles and low heels. 3 12-year-old girl, *c*. 1980. Cotton blouse with slashed neckline and wide cap sleeves, printed with tiger head and multicoloured leaves and flowers. Mid-calf-length straight-cut trousers with hip-level pockets and fly front fastening with button trim. Coloured Alice hair band. Heelless leather pumps with pointed toes. 4 5-year-old girl, *c*. 1980. Satin party dress, fitted bodice with contrast-colour shoulder-wide collar, trimmed with velvet ribbon bow on centre front, matching buttoned cuffs on long gathered sleeves, full skirt with wide knee-level frill. Hair worn in pony tail secured with coloured elastic band. Knitted cotton tights. Patent leather shoes with buttoned bar straps, leather soles and low heels. 5 5-year-old girl, *c*. 1980. Taffeta bridesmaid's dress, fitted bodice with curved panel seam, short puff sleeves and shoulder-wide contrast-colour satin frilled collar, matching wide sash with outsized bow at back and wide hair band. Knitted cotton tights. Satin shoes to match colour of dress, T-straps with button fastenings, leather soles and low heels. 6 4-year-old boy, *c*. 1980. School uniform: single-breasted wool flannel jacket with brass buttons, long sleeves, narrow collar and revers, three patch pockets, breast pocket with school emblem; wool flannel shorts; cotton flannel shirt worn with wool tie. Peaked cap with school emblem on front of sectioned crown. Knee-length knitted wool socks. Leather sandals with buckled T-straps, round toes and low heels. 7 12-year-old boy, *c*. 1981. Machine-knitted sleeveless sweater with all-over diamond pattern, edge of V-neck, armholes and hip-level rib in contrast colour. Fine wool shirt with small collar, long sleeves gathered into narrow cuffs. Straight-cut wool tweed trousers with hip-level pockets, fly front and central creases. Slip-on leather shoes with apron fronts, pointed toes and low heels.

1982 –1983

1 12-year-old girl, *c*. 1982. Patterned cotton dress, fitted bodice with asymmetric toggle button fastening, edges bound in contrast colour, matching edges of stand collar and short sleeves, knee-length box-pleat skirt. Hair worn in single braid and tied with ribbon bow. Knitted cotton tights. Leather pumps with round toes and low heels. 2 4-year-old boy, *c*. 1982. Hand-knitted sweater patterned with a row of elephants around the middle, high round neckline, full-length raglan sleeves with turned-back cuffs and ribbed hemline. Cotton cord trousers with straight-cut legs. Lace-up leather shoes with apron fronts, round toes and low heels. 3 5-year-old girl, *c*. 1983. Cotton shift dress with high yoke seam, front button fastening, mid-calf-length frilled hemline, contrast-colour Peter Pan collar, matching buttoned cuffs on full sleeves. Straw hat with wide brim. Leather sandals with buckled T-straps, round toes and low heels. 4 8-year-old girl, *c*. 1983. Knee-length smock dress, contrast-colour yoke with button fastening, self-fabric frilled edge, matching frill around high neckline and detail on cuffs of long sleeves. Straw hat, wide brim and high crown with draped band, matching dress fabric. Knitted cotton tights. Leather shoes with buttoned bar straps, round toes and low heels. 5 6-year-old girl, *c*. 1983. Striped knitted cotton dress with slashed neckline, plain knitted cotton collar with frilled edge, short sleeves, hip-length bodice with two-tier frilled skirt. Hair worn in bunches and tied with ribbons. Leather shoes with decorative bar straps above round toes, leather soles and low heels. 6 6-year-old girl, *c*. 1983. Knee-length spotted plastic raincoat, hood with drawstring tie under chin, high yoke with button fastening, long sleeves and low-set patch pockets. Ribbed cotton tights. Spotted plastic Wellington boots with round toes and combined rubber soles and heels. 7 4-year-old girl, *c*. 1982. Edge-to-edge wool waistcoat bound with contrast colour. Cotton blouse, high round neckline with pleated edge, matching cuffs on long sleeves, tucked bodice on either side of front buttoned strap fastening, worn with velvet ribbon bow tie at throat. Knee-length knife-pleated wool skirt with shoulder straps. Coloured Alice hair band. Knee-length knitted cotton socks. Leather slip-on shoes with apron fronts and round toes.

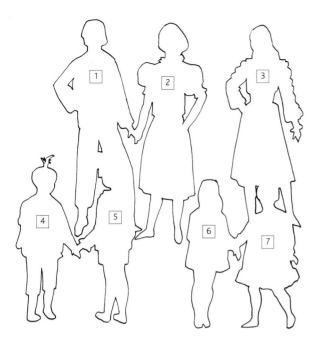

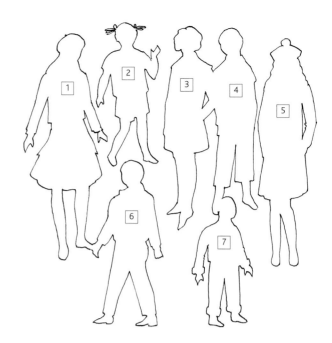

1984 –1986

1 12-year-old girl, *c.* 1984. Two-piece brushed cotton track suit: collarless top with centre-front zip fastening, two hip-level curved patch pockets, full-length raglan sleeves gathered into knitted cuffs, matching finish around neckline and hemlines of top and loose-fitting trousers. Lace-up trainers. 2 12-year-old girl, *c.* 1985. Collarless single-breasted suede waistcoat with cut-away armholes, two small patch pockets above pointed hemline. Cotton satin blouse with frilled neckline, matching narrow cuffs on short puff sleeves, pin tucks on either side of centre-front button strap fastening. Below-knee-length taffeta skirt gathered from under wide waistband. Flesh-coloured nylon tights. Leather pumps with low vamps, round toes and low heels. 3 12-year-old girl, *c.* 1986. Cotton blouse with shoulder-wide curved yoke edged with frill of self-fabric and trimmed with lace, matching stand collar, full sleeves, sleeve cuffs and tucked bodice. Below-knee-length skirt gathered from under wide waistband, trimmed with lace to match blouse. Flesh-coloured nylon tights. Leather shoes with decorative straps, pointed toes and low heels. 4 4-year-old girl, *c.* 1985. Hip-length wool jacket with small collar, long sleeves with stitched cuffs and drawstring hem. Mid-calf-length cotton trousers. Backpack in form of large teddy bear. Hair worn in pony tail on top of head, secured with elastic band. Leather sandals with wide straps and thick cork combined soles and heels. 5 6-year-old girl, *c.* 1984. Hip-length knitted wool sweater, long sleeves with ribbed cuffs, matching neckline and hemline. Mini-length straight skirt in matching wool. Acrylic blouse with frilled neckline and cuffs. Hair bound with scarf tied into large bow. Knitted wool tights. Heelless leather pumps with round toes. 6 4-year-old girl, *c.* 1986. Mini-length flared wool jersey dress, high round neckline bound with contrast colour, matching stripes on short sleeves and upper bodice, skirt in second contrast colour. Wide coloured Alice hair band. Knitted wool tights. Leather shoes with buttoned bar straps and round toes. 7 4-year-old girl, *c.* 1986. Mini-length striped cotton satin shift dress with gathers from shoulder yoke, long sleeves gathered into buttoned cuffs, deep frill around hemline, detachable contrast-colour collar with spotted silk scarf. Knitted cotton tights. Leather shoes with decorative straps, round toes and low heels.

1987 –1988

1 10-year-old girl, *c.* 1988. Edge-to-edge hip-length floral print jacket with shirt collar and full-length sleeves. Floral print fine wool blouse with button fastening from under shirt collar and long sleeves. Knee-length checked wool gathered skirt, worn with floral print fine wool overskirt with pointed hemline. Wool beret with central stalk. Knitted wool tights. Leather pumps with low-cut vamps, round toes and low heels. 2 3-year-old girl, *c.* 1987. Holiday wear: cotton blouse with printed stripes and central motif, high round neckline, button fastenings on shoulders, short sleeves and drawstring waist; cotton shorts. Hair worn in bunches and tied with ribbon bows. Heelless plastic shoes with buttoned bar straps and round toes. 3 5-year-old girl, *c.* 1988. Holiday wear: mini-length cotton shift dress, hip-length sleeveless bodice with shoulder-wide sailor collar bound with contrast colour, matching centre-front bow, armholes and seam above flared skirt. Leather shoes with wide buttoned bar straps, round toes and low heels. 4 5-year-old boy, *c.* 1987. Beachwear: two-piece playsuit consisting of hip-length striped knitted cotton top with short sleeves and contrast-colour Peter Pan collar above buttoned strap fastening; mid-calf-length trousers in matching fabric. Coloured lace-up trainers. 5 8-year-old girl, *c.* 1987. Hand-knitted wool sweater with geometric pattern in contrast colour under ribbed high neckline, ribbing repeated on cuffs of long sleeves and hemline. Checked wool mini skirt with hip-level pockets. Hand-knitted wool beret with contrast-colour pompon on top. Knitted wool tights. Leather shoes with apron fronts and round toes. 6 6-year-old boy, *c.* 1987. Waist-length cotton denim jacket with personalized logo on back, shirt collar, long sleeves with cuffs with press-stud fasteners, fastenings repeated on adjustable waistband, top-stitched edges and detail. Cotton denim jeans with side hip pockets, patch pockets with press-stud flaps on either side at back, top-stitched edges and seams. Brightly coloured knitted cotton socks. Lace-up leather shoes with rubber soles and heels. 7 4-year-old boy, *c.* 1987. Short edge-to-edge cotton jacket with button trim, collar and revers, long sleeves with turned-back cuffs to reveal striped lining. Knitted cotton T-shirt with high round neckline. Checked cotton trousers, straight-cut legs with wide turn-ups, deep waistband with button fastening and fly front. Brightly coloured knitted cotton socks. Leather-look lace-up shoes with apron fronts and combined soles and low heels.

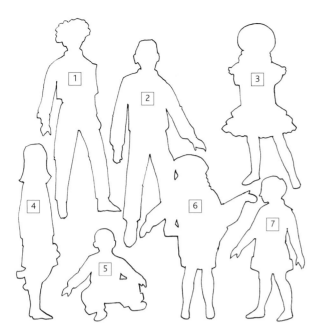

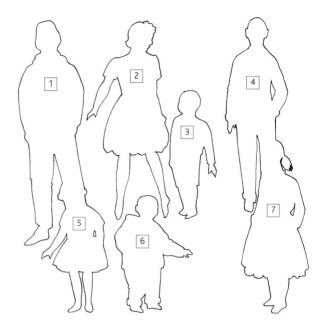

1989–1990

1 10-year-old girl, *c.* 1990. Waist-length cotton denim jacket with shirt-style pointed collar, single-breasted press-stud fastening, matching cuffs on long sleeves and flaps on patch pockets, top-stitched edges and detail. Multicoloured striped knitted cotton T-shirt with high round neckline and long sleeves. Cotton denim jeans with narrow legs, fly fronts, side-hip pockets, top-stitched edges and detail. Multicoloured silk scarf worn tied around head. Knitted cotton socks. Lace-up canvas shoes with combined rubber soles and heels. 2 12-year-old boy, *c.* 1990. Two-piece knitted cotton sports suit: top bloused onto contrast-colour hip band, matching yoke, collar with centre-front zip fastening, patches on inside of upper sleeves and elasticated cuffs at wrist level; loose-fitting trousers gathered into elastic on waist and into elasticated cuffs at ankle level. Knitted cotton T-shirt with high round neck and long sleeves. Multicoloured peaked cap. Lace-up trainers with combined rubber soles and heels. 3 4-year-old girl, *c.* 1989. Cotton dress with centre-front button fastening from under high round neckline to low waistline, short sleeves with frilled hem, matching short three-tier frilled skirt. Straw hat with wide turned-back brim. Spotted nylon tights. Heelless leather sandals with buckled T-straps and openwork above round toes. 4 6-year-old girl, *c.* 1989. Knitted cotton shirt top with contrast-colour shirt-style collar and buttoned bar strap fastening, matching sewn cuffs on short sleeves and hip-level band. Short flared cotton denim skirt. Knitted ribbed wool tights. Leather shoes with buttoned bar straps, round toes and low heels. 5 1-year-old boy, *c.* 1990. Striped cotton dungarees, bib front with adjustable shoulder straps, inset waistband, trousers with wide legs and deep turned-back cuffs. Cotton denim shirt with large pointed collar and long sleeves with buttoned cuffs, top-stitched edges and detail. Knitted cotton socks. Two-colour lace-up heelless leather boots with round toes. 6 5-year-old girl, *c.* 1989. Knee-length hand-knitted wool sweater dress with high polo neck, wide raglan sleeves with stripes of pattern at wrist, matching detail above hem of knee-length tight skirt. Wide stiffened cloth headband with gathered-on hand-knitted crown, trimmed with large pompon on one side. Short hand-knitted wool mittens. Knitted wool tights. Multicoloured lace-up canvas trainers with round rubber toecaps. 7 4-year-old boy, *c.* 1990. Cotton denim playsuit with centre-front press-stud fastening, wide shoulder straps, pin-tucked detail on either side of front bodice, shorts with wide legs and deep top-stitched turned-back cuffs. Spotted cotton neck scarf knotted at front. Lace-up canvas trainers with high tongues, round toecaps, combined soles and heels.

1991–1992

1 12-year-old boy, *c.* 1991. Waist-length wool hooded jacket with centre-front zip fastening, full-length sleeves gathered into cuffs, zipped pockets in sleeves and above waistband on either side front of jacket. Knitted cotton polo shirt. Straight-cut trousers gathered into cuffs at ankle level, hip-level pockets, leather patch pockets with flaps or zips. Brimless knitted cotton pull-on hat. Lace-up trainers with combined soles and heels. 2 6-year-old girl, *c.* 1992. Bridesmaid's outfit: star-patterned silk taffeta dress, fitted bodice with button fastening from under high round neckline, short sleeves, knee-length puff-ball skirt. Pleated and gathered headdress in matching fabric. Knitted cotton tights. Satin shoes with buttoned bar straps, round toes, leather soles and low heels. 3 3-year-old boy, *c.* 1992. Pageboy suit: single-breasted silk brocade jacket with narrow stand collar and long sleeves; knee-length velvet breeches with brass button detail on outside seam above hemline. Knitted cotton tights. Leather shoes with buckle above high tongue, round toes and low heels. 4 10-year-old boy, *c.* 1991. Machine-knitted wool collarless single-breasted cardigan with all-over multicolour pattern, fastening with leather buttons through contrast-colour ribbed edge, matching cuffs on long sleeves and hemline. Cotton shirt with buttoned-down collar. Straight-cut cotton cord trousers with side hip pockets, central creases and turn-ups. Lace-up leather-look shoes with apron fronts and round toes. 5 5-year-old girl, *c.* 1991. Summer school uniform: striped cotton pinafore dress, bib front with buttoned shoulder straps, inset waistband with button fastening on one side, knee-length gathered skirt. Cotton blouse with wide collar, front button fastening and short sleeves with sewn cuffs. Straw hat with domed crown and narrow turned-back brim. Knee-length knitted cotton socks. Leather sandals with buckled T-straps, openwork detail above round toes, leather soles and low heels. 6 3-year-old boy, *c.* 1992. Padded waterproof hooded jacket with concealed centre-front zip fastening under buttoned strap, long sleeves gathered into elasticated cuffs, patch pockets with buttoned flaps, on either side of centre front, drawstring hem, top-stitched edges and detail. Cotton T-shirt with high round neckline. Cotton denim jeans with rollback hems. Coloured knitted wool socks. Slip-on leather-look shoes with Velcro strap fastenings over apron fronts, leather soles and low heels. 7 7-year-old girl, *c.* 1991. Cotton blouse with button fastening under frilled collar, matching cuffs on long sleeves. Knee-length striped cotton gathered skirt with elasticated waist, wide shoulder straps and outsized patch pockets, skirt worn over visible lace-edged petticoat. Knitted cotton tights. Leather sandals with buckled T-straps and openwork above round toes, leather soles and low heels.

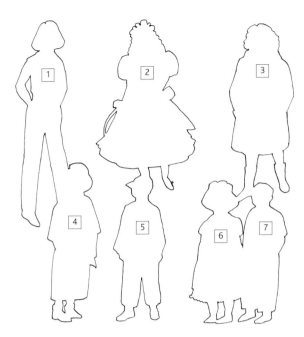

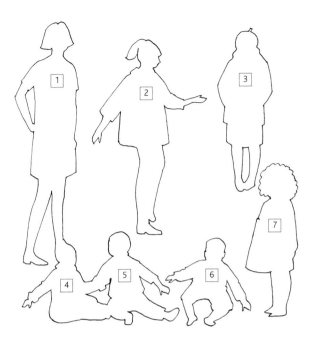

1993 –1995

1 8-year-old girl, *c.* 1995. Sleeveless cotton denim blouse with front buttoned strap fastening under shirt-style collar, shaped yoke, large patch pockets with buttoned flaps and inverted box-pleats on either side of centre front, contrast-colour top-stitched edges and detail. Narrow-cut cotton denim jeans with embroidered detail under hip-level pockets, fly front fastening, top-stitched edges and detail, jeans worn with metal-buckled wide leather belt. Lace-up canvas shoes with gingham-effect panel above toecaps, thick soles and low heels. 2 8-year-old girl, *c.* 1994. Bridesmaid's outfit: floral patterned silk dress, fitted panelled bodice with sweetheart neckline and outsized puff sleeves gathered into wide cuffs, full skirt ruched and secured with silk flowers on side seams, centre front and centre back and edged with wide border of lace; stiffened plain silk underskirt, matching large bow and tails at back. Headdress of silk flowers and leaves. Knitted cotton tights. Silk pumps with bow trim above round toes, leather soles and low heels. 3 8-year-old girl, *c.* 1994. Fake fur coat printed with stylized sheep, concealed front fastening from under large collar to knee-length hemline, long sleeves and hip-level welt pockets. Stretch fabric hair band. Mid-calf-length plastic Wellington boots with round toes and combined soles and low heels. 4 5-year-old boy, *c.* 1994. Cotton denim overalls, bib front with large patch pocket, half with press-studded flap, adjustable straps, belt carriers above waist seam, mid-calf-length trousers with hip-length pockets and fly front fastening, top-stitched edges and detail. Collarless striped cotton shirt with dropped shoulderline and elbow-length sleeves. Unstructured cotton denim hat with tall crown and wide brim. Knitted wool socks rolled over lace-up leather boots with round toes and low heels. 5 4-year-old boy, *c.* 1993. Broad striped knitted cotton sweatshirt with high round neckline, dropped shoulderline, long sleeves and logo on centre of chest. Wide knitted cotton trousers elasticated around ankles. Striped cotton peaked baseball cap. Two-tone lace-up trainers with high tongues, combined soles and heels. 6 4-year-old girl, *c.* 1995. High-waist cotton dress with high yoke seam, short sleeves, contrast-fabric collar, matching buttoned strap fastening and hip-level patch and flap pockets. Cotton underdress with long sleeves and frill-trimmed hemline. Velvet hat with large ruched crown and wide turned-back brim. Plastic sandals with buckled T-straps and strap front, moulded soles and low heels. 7 3-year-old boy, *c.* 1995. Striped cotton overalls, bib front with large patch pocket, buttoned straps, buttoned side-opening and wide legs. Knitted cotton T-shirt with round neckline and short sleeves. Cotton baseball cap with large peak. Two-tone lace-up trainers.

1996 –1999

1 12-year-old girl, *c.* 1997. Pony print cotton two-piece suit: sleeveless single-breasted unfitted jacket with low collarless neckline; mini-length skirt in matching fabric. Knitted cotton T-shirt with V-neckline and short sleeves. Knitted cotton tights. Leather-look shoes with low vamps above round toes, platform soles and thick heels. 2 8-year-old girl, *c.* 1996. Floral print unfitted cotton top with contrast-colour collar and three-quarter-length sleeves. Hair worn in pony tail secured with coloured elastic band. Striped knitted wool tights. Leather sandals with open toes, high vamps and sling-back straps, platform soles and low heels. 3 4-year-old girl, *c.* 1998. Wool jersey two-piece suit: hooded jacket with centre-front zip fastening and long sleeves with turned-back cuffs showing lining; knee-length straight skirt in matching fabric. Knitted cotton T-shirt with high round neckline bound in contrast colour. Pull-on two-tone knitted wool hat with looped stalk in middle of crown. Striped knitted wool tights. Leather shoes with double bar straps above round toes. 4 Baby, *c.* 1996. Brushed cotton collarless playsuit with centre-front Velcro fastening, long sleeves and mid-calf-length trousers gathered into stretch cuffs. Striped cotton blouse with long sleeves, turned back on wrists, contrast-colour collar. Two-tone brushed cotton bonnet with point on crown and embroidered rabbit on either side, Velcro fastening under chin. Striped knitted cotton socks. 5 Baby, *c.* 1997. Single-breasted striped sleeveless cotton waistcoat, fastening with large buttons, mock welt pockets on either side. Patterned brushed cotton sleeveless playsuit with front press-stud fastening under wide collarless neckline, ankle-length trousers. Striped cotton blouse, three-quarter-length sleeves with contrast-colour cuffs, matching Peter Pan collar. Pull-on knitted cotton multicoloured striped hat. Heelless soft leather boots. 6 Baby, *c.* 1999. Checked cotton gingham overalls with adjustable straps and knee-length trousers with turned-back cuffs. Knitted cotton shirt with high round neckline and long sleeves with cuffs. Cotton hat with crown gathered onto wide stiffened band. Short knitted cotton socks. Lace-up trainers with contrast-colour combined soles and heels. 7 5-year-old girl, *c.* 1998. Hand-knitted sleeveless wool pinafore dress with large pocket under low neckline, border of flowers around hem of knee-length flared skirt, flower repeated on pocket. Hand-knitted wool sweater with high round neckline and three-quarter-length cuffed sleeves. Short knitted wool socks. Ankle-length lace-up leather boots with round toecaps and stacked heels.

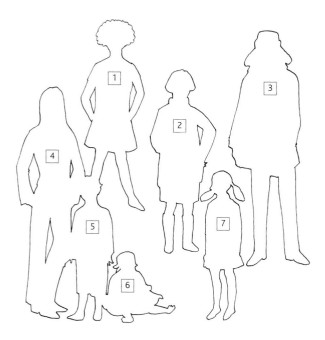

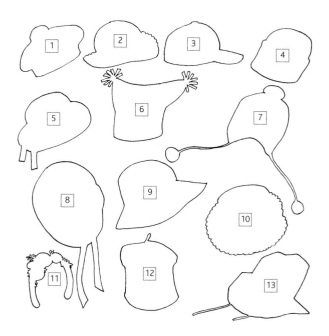

2000 – Present Day

1 6-year-old girl, *c.* 2008. Knitted cotton T-shirt with high round neckline bound in contrast colour, matching short sleeves and hemline, main body printed with large butterfly and border of flowers around hemline. Mini-length cotton denim skirt with two patch pockets above inverted pleats, top-stitched edges and detail. Knitted stretch cotton tights with multicoloured stripes and stylized flowers. Heelless leather shoes with Velcro strap fastenings above round toes. 2 6-year-old girl, *c.* 2006. Machine-knitted wool dress with ribbed polo neck, matching ribbed cuffs on long sleeves and hemline of narrow skirt, horizontal multicolour striped panel gathered from high waist seam and into seam above hemline. Ribbed knitted wool tights. Mid-calf-length plastic Wellington boots decorated with stars, combined soles and heels. 3 12-year-old boy, *c.* 2008. Padded waterproof parka coat with faux fur-trimmed collar, centre-front zip fastening under buttoned strap, long raglan sleeves with adjustable buttoned straps above top-stitched cuffs, matching top-stitching on hip-level patch and flap pockets, diagonal chest-level welt pockets, waist-level jetted pockets and edges and seams. Knitted cotton T-shirt with high round neckline and personalized logo on centre of chest. Straight-cut cotton denim jeans. Pull-on stretch wool hat with turned-back cuff. Leather-look shoes with Velcro strap fastening, thick soles and heels. 4 12-year-old girl, *c.* 2000. Short brushed cotton hooded jacket with centre-front zip fastening through large patch pocket with openings on either side, contrast-colour long flared sleeves with inset band of self-colour on upper arms. Waist-length knitted cotton T-shirt with high round neckline. Hipster cotton denim jeans with side hip pockets, fly front fastening, top-stitched edges and detail. Leather-look shoes with Velcro strap fastenings, thick soles and heels. 5 4-year-old boy, *c.* 2007. Single-breasted linen-look sleeveless waistcoat, fastening with large buttons, waist-level diagonal welt pockets. Cotton shirt with narrow stand collar and long sleeves with buttoned cuffs. Mid-calf-length striped linen trousers. Lace-up leather shoes with acrylic soles and heels. 6 Baby, *c.* 2006. Floral print pinafore dress, bib front with buttoned straps, full skirt with split sides, finished with self-fabric rouleau bows. Patterned cotton muslin dress with Peter Pan collar, elbow-length sleeves gathered from dropped shoulderline and ending in frilled cuffs, full gathered skirt. Patterned cotton muslin hat, crown gathered on checked cotton gingham band. 7 6-year-old girl, *c.* 2002. Machine-knitted wool cardigan with centre-front zip fastening from under pointed collar to hip-level hemline, long sleeves with contrast-colour stripes from elbow to wrist, matching stripes on lower bodice. Striped knitted cotton T-shirt with high round neckline. Mini-length flared wool skirt. Hair worn in bunches and secured with coloured elastic bands. Knitted wool tights. Trainers with contrast-colour laces.

Hats 1983 – Present Day

1 8-year-old girl, *c.* 1983. Machine-knitted hat with unstructured crown gathered onto stiffened band, pompon trim in centre of crown. 2 2-year-old girl, *c.* 1999. Patterned cotton hat with large sectioned crown and wide brim turned up at front, edged with self-fabric frill and embroidered with flower motif on front. 3 9-year-old boy, *c.* 1995. Cotton denim cap, sectioned crown with button trim on top, embroidered logo above stiffened peak, top-stitched edges and detail. 4 6-year-old boy, *c.* 1997. Hand-knitted pull-on hat, unstructured crown and turned-back cuff with felt name initial in centre. 5 6-year-old girl, *c.* 1992. School uniform straw hat with narrow turned-back brim, tall crown with ribbon band and trailing ends. 6 4-year-old boy, *c.* 2006. Machine-knitted wool pull-on hat, multicolour striped rectangle with tassel trim on two corners. 7 18-month-old boy, *c.* 2005. Hand-knitted angora wool bonnet, close-fitting over ears, fastening with knitted ties under chin, pompon on each end, matching trim on centre of crown. 8 10-year-old girl, *c.* 1985. Straw hat with wide flat brim edged with fancy braid and ribbon, matching band and trailing ends on shallow crown. 9 3-year-old girl, *c.* 2001. Floral print cotton sun hat with tall sectioned crown, wide unstructured brim, top-stitched edges and detail. 10 3-year-old girl, *c.* 2006. Floral print cotton velvet hat, tall crown with self-fabric band trimmed with ribbon edged with lace frill, matching edge of wide unstructured brim. 11 6-year-old girl, *c.* 1994. Bridesmaid's headdress: silk-covered hair band trimmed on front with silk flowers and leaves. 12 5-year-old girl, *c.* 1998. Machine-knitted pull-on hat, tall unstructured crown with single loop on top and decorated with bands of contrast-colour stripes. 13 6-year-old girl, *c.* 2007. Unstructured spotted cotton sun hat with tall crown and wide brim turned up at front, rouleau ties under chin.

Chart from Antiquity to 1799

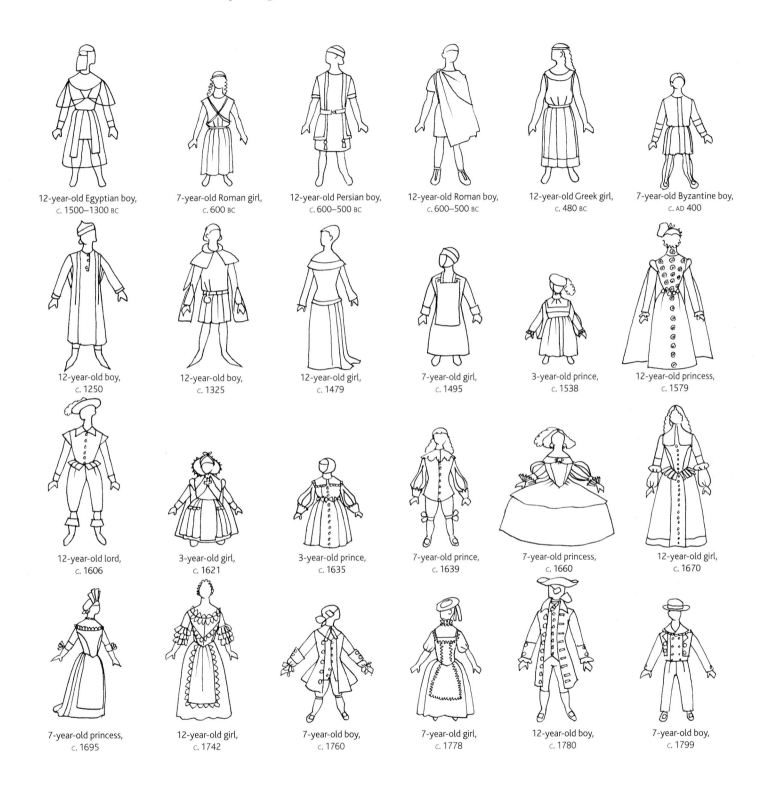

12-year-old Egyptian boy,
c. 1500–1300 BC

7-year-old Roman girl,
c. 600 BC

12-year-old Persian boy,
c. 600–500 BC

12-year-old Roman boy,
c. 600–500 BC

12-year-old Greek girl,
c. 480 BC

7-year-old Byzantine boy,
c. AD 400

12-year-old boy,
c. 1250

12-year-old boy,
c. 1325

12-year-old girl,
c. 1479

7-year-old girl,
c. 1495

3-year-old prince,
c. 1538

12-year-old princess,
c. 1579

12-year-old lord,
c. 1606

3-year-old girl,
c. 1621

3-year-old prince,
c. 1635

7-year-old prince,
c. 1639

7-year-old princess,
c. 1660

12-year-old girl,
c. 1670

7-year-old princess,
c. 1695

12-year-old girl,
c. 1742

7-year-old boy,
c. 1760

7-year-old girl,
c. 1778

12-year-old boy,
c. 1780

7-year-old boy,
c. 1799

Chart from 1800 to 1849

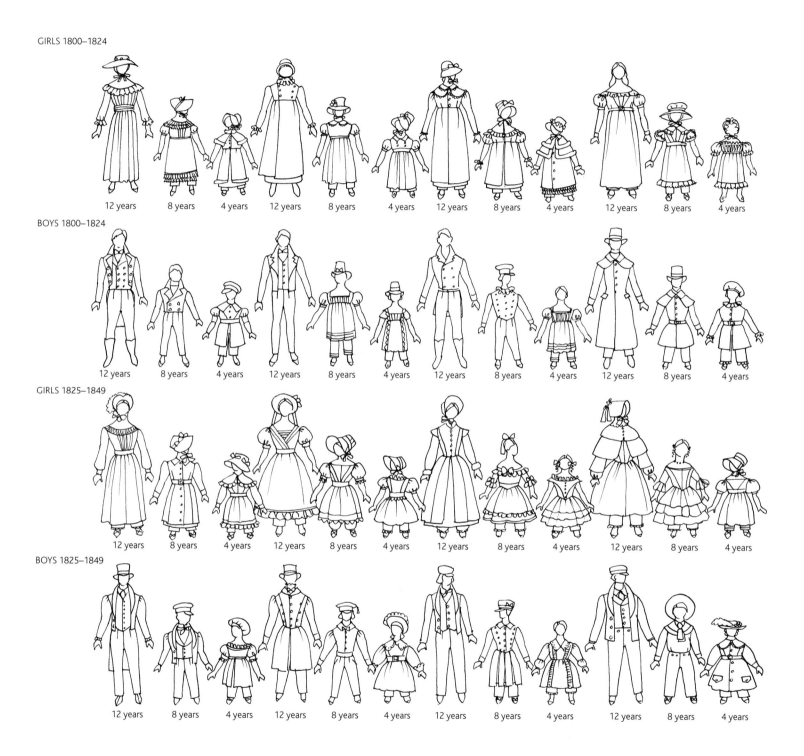

GIRLS 1800–1824

12 years   8 years   4 years   12 years   8 years   4 years   12 years   8 years   4 years   12 years   8 years   4 years

BOYS 1800–1824

12 years   8 years   4 years   12 years   8 years   4 years   12 years   8 years   4 years   12 years   8 years   4 years

GIRLS 1825–1849

12 years   8 years   4 years   12 years   8 years   4 years   12 years   8 years   4 years   12 years   8 years   4 years

BOYS 1825–1849

12 years   8 years   4 years   12 years   8 years   4 years   12 years   8 years   4 years   12 years   8 years   4 years

Chart from 1850 to 1899

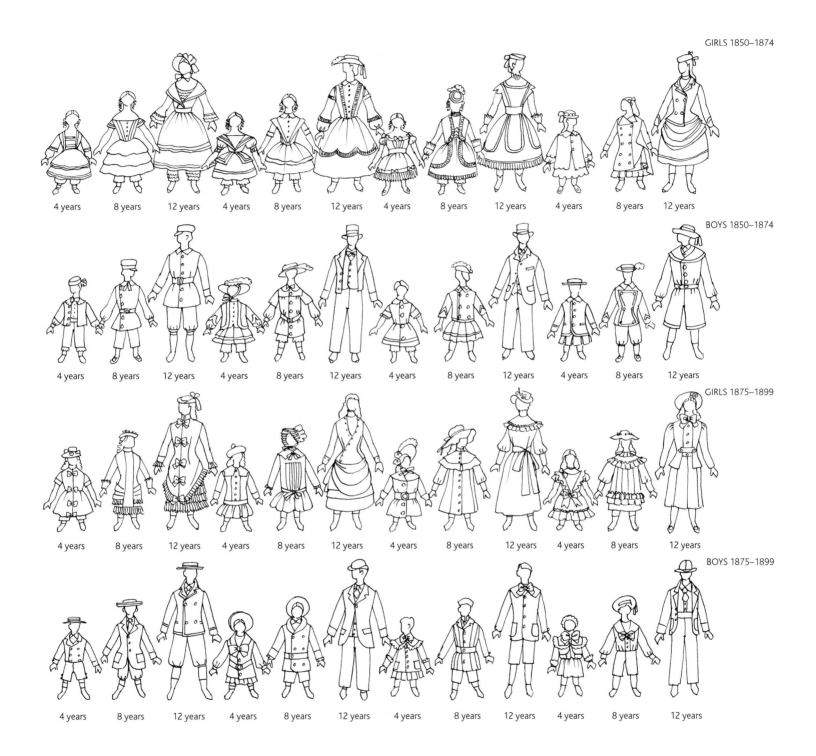

GIRLS 1850–1874

4 years   8 years   12 years   4 years   8 years   12 years   4 years   8 years   12 years   4 years   8 years   12 years

BOYS 1850–1874

4 years   8 years   12 years   4 years   8 years   12 years   4 years   8 years   12 years   4 years   8 years   12 years

GIRLS 1875–1899

4 years   8 years   12 years   4 years   8 years   12 years   4 years   8 years   12 years   4 years   8 years   12 years

BOYS 1875–1899

4 years   8 years   12 years   4 years   8 years   12 years   4 years   8 years   12 years   4 years   8 years   12 years

Chart from 1900 to 1949

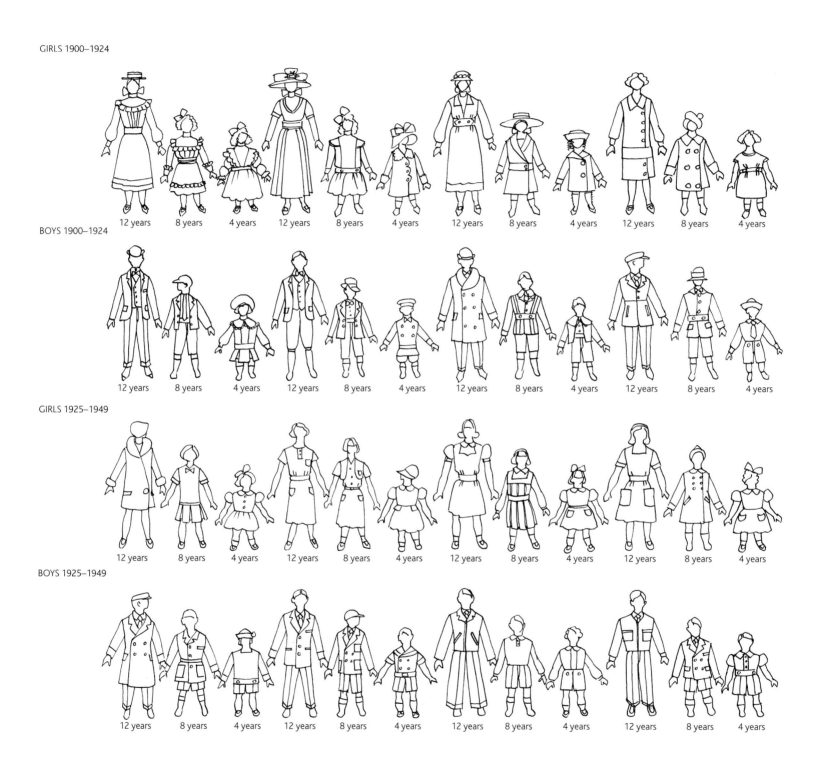

GIRLS 1900–1924

12 years 8 years 4 years 12 years 8 years 4 years 12 years 8 years 4 years 12 years 8 years 4 years

BOYS 1900–1924

12 years 8 years 4 years 12 years 8 years 4 years 12 years 8 years 4 years 12 years 8 years 4 years

GIRLS 1925–1949

12 years 8 years 4 years 12 years 8 years 4 years 12 years 8 years 4 years 12 years 8 years 4 years

BOYS 1925–1949

12 years 8 years 4 years 12 years 8 years 4 years 12 years 8 years 4 years 12 years 8 years 4 years

Chart from 1950 to Present Day

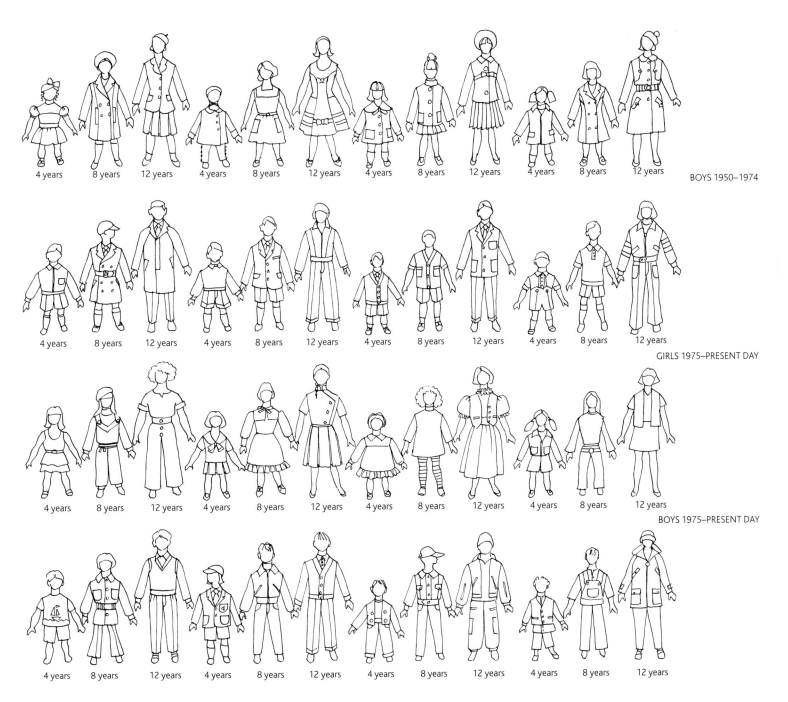

4 years 8 years 12 years 4 years 8 years 12 years 4 years 8 years 12 years 4 years 8 years 12 years

Sources for Children's Costume

Anderson Black, J., and Madge Garland, *A History of Fashion*, London 1975

Ashleford, Jane, *Dress in the Age of Elizabeth I*, London 1988

Birbari, Elizabeth, *Dress in Italian Painting: 1460–1500*, London 1975

Blum, Stella, *Fashions and Costumes from Godey's Lady's Book*, New York 1985

Boucher, François, *A History of Costume in the West*, London 1965

Bradfield, Nancy, *Historical Costumes of England from the Eleventh to the Twentieth Century*, London 1958

———, *Costume in Detail: Women's Dress 1730–1930*, London 1968

Brooke, Iris, *English Children's Costume 1775–1920*, London 1930

———, *A History of English Costume*, London 1937

———, *English Costume of the Early Middle Ages: The Tenth to the Thirteenth Centuries*, London 1948

———, *English Costume of the Later Middle Ages: The Fourteenth and Fifteenth Centuries*, London 1948

———, *English Costume in the Age of Elizabeth: The Sixteenth Century*, London 1948

———, *English Costume of the Seventeenth Century*, London 1948

———, *English Costume of the Nineteenth Century*, London 1948

Brooke, Iris, and James Laver, *English Costume of the Eighteenth Century*, London 1949

Buck, Anne, *Clothes and the Child: A Handbook of Children's Dress in England 1500–1900*, Bedford 1996

Carnegy, Vicky, *Fashions of a Decade: The 1980s*, London 1990

Contini, Mila, *Fashion: From Ancient Egypt to the Present Day*, London 1965

Cunnington, C. Willett, *English Women's Clothing in the Present Century*, London 1952

Cunnington, C. Willett, and Phillis Cunnington, *Handbook of Mediaeval Costume*, London 1952

———, *Handbook of English Costume in the Seventeenth Century*, London 1955

———, *Handbook of English Costume in the Nineteenth Century*, London 1959

———, *Handbook of English Costume in the Eighteenth Century*, London 1972

Cunnington, C. Willett, Phillis Cunnington and Charles Beard, *A Dictionary of English Costume*, London 1974

Cunnington, Phillis, and Anne Buck, *Children's Costume in England: From the Fourteenth to the End of the Nineteenth Century*, London 1972

Dorner, Jane, *Fashion in the Twenties and Thirties*, London 1973

———, *Fashion in the Forties and Fifties*, London 1975

Ewing, Elizabeth, *History of Children's Costume*, London 1977

Fowler, Kenneth, *The Age of Plantagenet and Valois*, London 1980

Gaunt, William, *Court Painting in England from Tudor to Victorian Times*, London 1980

Ginsburg, Madeleine, *Victorian Dress in Photographs*, London 1982

Gorsline, Douglas, *What People Wore: A Visual History of Dress from Ancient Times to the Twentieth Century*, London 1978

Hansen, Henny Harald, *Costume Cavalcade*, London 1956

Harris, Carol, and Mike Brown, *Children's Costumes*, New York 2002

Harris, Kristina, *The Child in Fashion 1750–1920*, Atglen 1999

Hartley, Dorothy, *Mediaeval Costume and Life*, London 1931

Herald, Jacqueline, *Renaissance Dress in Italy 1400–1500*, London 1981

Holland, Vyvyan, *Hand Coloured Fashion Plates 1770–1899*, London 1988

Houston, Mary G., *Ancient Greek, Roman and Byzantine Costume and Decorations*, London 1930

———, *European Costume from the Thirteenth Century to the Commencement of the Seventeenth Century with Decorations*, London 1930

———, *Medieval Costume in England and France: The 13th, 14th and 15th Centuries*, London 1939

Houston, Mary G., and Florence S. Hornblower, *Ancient Egyptian, Assyrian and Persian Costume and Decorations*, London 1920

Langdon, Helen, *Everyday Life in Painting*, Oxford 1979

Langley Moore, Doris, *The Child in Fashion*, London 1953

Laver, James, *Children's Fashions in the Nineteenth Century*, London 1951

———, *Costume Through the Ages*, London 1963

———, *Costume in Antiquity*, London 1964

———, *A Concise History of Costume*, London 1969

MacPhail, Anna, *The Well Dressed Child: Children's Clothing 1820–1940*, Atglen 1999

Schorsch, Anita, *Images of Childhood: An Illustrated Social History*, New York 1979

Stevenson, Pauline, *Edwardian Fashion*, London 1980

Villa, Nora, *Children in their Party Dress*, Modena 1989

Waller, Jane (ed.), *Some Things for the Children*, London 1974

Wilcox, R. Turner, *Five Centuries of American Costume*, New York 1963

———, *The Dictionary of Costume*, New York 1970

Yarwood, Doreen, *English Costume: From the Second Century BC to 1967*, London 1967

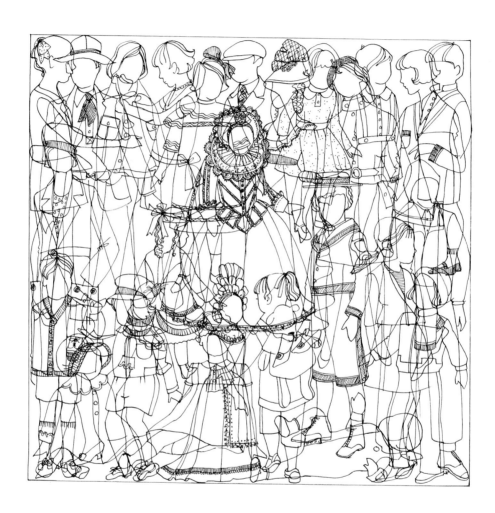